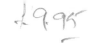

Basic
Human
Embryology

C P Wendell Smith
MB, BS, PH D (LOND), DOBST RCOG, MACE, FRACOG
Professor of Anatomy, University of Tasmania, Formerly Associate Professor of Anatomy, University of New South Wales, Formerly Lecturer in Anatomy, Guy's Hospital Medical School, University of London

P L Williams
MA, MB, B CHIR (CAMB), DSC (LOND)
Emeritus Professor of Anatomy, University of London, Formerly Professor of Anatomy at Guy's Hospital Medical School, University of London

Sylvia Treadgold
MSIAD, AIMBI, MAMI
Formerly Senior Medical Artist, Guy's Hospital Medical School, University of London and Addenbrooke's Hospital, Cambridge

Pitman

PITMAN PUBLISHING LIMITED
128 Long Acre, London WC2E 9AN

Associated Companies
Pitman Publishing Pty Ltd, Melbourne
Pitman Publishing New Zealand Ltd, Wellington

First published 1966
Second Edition 1969
ELBS Edition 1969
Polish Edition (Panstwowy Zaklad Wydawnictiv Lekarskich,
Warsaw) 1972
Italian Edition (Edi, Ermes s.r.l. Milan) 1976
Second Italian Edition 1981
Japanese Edition (Hirokawa Publishing Co, Tokyo) 1979
Third Edition 1984

British Library Cataloguing in Publication Data
Wendell Smith, C. P.
  Basic human embryology
  1. Embryology, Human
  I. Title   II. Williams, Peter L.
  III. Treadgold, Sylvia
  611'. 013   QM602

ISBN 0 272 79720 0

© P L Williams, C P Wendell Smith and Sylvia Treadgold 1966,
1969, 1984

Text set in 8½/10 pt Linotron 202 Palatino,
printed and bound in Great Britain

Contents

Preface

The study of embryology provides a logical basis for topographical anatomy, an explanation—albeit superficial—of many congenital anomalies and a scaffolding for future studies in obstetrics and paediatrics. Most significantly, it provides an appropriate introduction to a more thorough treatment of those aspects of the life of cells and cell communities which lie at the heart of modern biology and at the core of medical science. It is thus regrettable that the study of embryology continues to be curtailed in or even absent from the curriculum of some medical schools.

We prepared this book because we believe embryology is important and that its essentials can be presented in small compass, if adequately illustrated. We have included sections designed to bridge the gap between prenatal development and obstetrics, paediatrics and adult anatomy. We have also included sections designed for orientation in general biology and comparative embryology. Within each system, organogenesis is generally dealt with in chronological sequence but details of times are not given. Instead, a chronological summary of some key features of prenatal organogenesis, with a discussion of teratogenesis, is included in the appendix.

In preparing this third edition the whole text has been reviewed and updated. Although originally aimed at students of medicine and dentistry, the book has also been used by those studying for higher professional examinations, by medical ancillaries and by others. In response to requests from users of the second edition, we have included simple introductions before each major section, to give perspective and to set the stage, while after each section we have dealt with the common congenital anomalies in greater detail than previously. For the same reason we have included a concise treatment of human genetics as applied to the individual and of aberrations of developmental mechanisms.

We have again followed the principle of illustrating what can be illustrated and using the text to stress points and to convey what cannot be illustrated. The illustrations thus provide on the one hand a treatment intermediate between the new introductions and the general text, and on the other hand a means of rapid revision. All are diagrammatic with varying degrees of realism. We believe that the place for photomicrographs and actual sections is in a parallel practical course. Diagrams and related texts are usually presented on the same double-page spread, which facilitates reading and removes the need for many figure and cross-references. The index should be used to locate discussion or illustration of a particular item.

The prime responsibility for this edition has rested with one of us (CPWS) because of the involvement of the other (PLW) in the production of successive editions of *Gray's Anatomy*. As a result of that involvement, the treatment in the two books is complementary. In this book we have attempted to summarize the current state of knowledge and, on occasion, to make informed guesses which go beyond this—a technique which kept the second edition up to date for many years after publication. In *Gray* there is an expanded treatment of some aspects, including historical perspective, cytogenesis, histogenesis and references to which the reader is referred.* The few additional references used in the preparation of this edition are listed below. Most of them will be included in the 37th edition of *Gray*, currently in preparation.

All the illustrations are the work of Sylvia Treadgold who conceived the idea of the book after attending the embryology lectures given by one of us (PLW). Miss Treadgold, a medical illustrator of international repute, was then Senior Medical Artist to Guy's Hospital Medical School where the foundations of the book were laid. We count ourselves fortunate in having had her collaboration throughout the project. The other author became involved and the project was started when, as a result of the desirable practice then followed of rotating responsibilities, he began to give the course.

We regard it as significant that both this book and recent editions of *Gray* have come from the same stable in a period when the Department of Anatomy has been headed by our colleague and friend, Roger Warwick, and we thank him for his encouragement. We would also like to thank our other colleagues of the Departments of Anatomy, Guy's Hospital Medical School, and the University of Tasmania, and our wives for their advice, active help, support and constructive criticism. Mrs Irene Williams typed much of the manuscript of the first edition. We regret the death of Mrs Margaret Hesketh (née Kellick) who typed the balance at the University of New South Wales. For the typing and much of the organizing of this edition we thank Mrs Margaret Martyn and Mrs Margaret Galbraith of the University of Tasmania.

Colin Wendell Smith *and* Peter L. Williams

* Williams, P L and Warwick, R (Eds) (1980) *Gray's Anatomy*, 36th edition. Churchill Livingstone, Edinburgh.

Additional References

Afzelius, B (1979) The immotile-cilia syndrome and other ciliary diseases. *International Review of Experimental Pathology*, **19**, 1–43.

Ellis, R W B (1947) 'Introduction' *Child Health and Development*, J and A Churchill Ltd, London.

Ford, E B (1940) Polymorphism and taxonomy. In *The New Systematics* (Ed. Huxley, J S). The Clarendon Press, Oxford.

Hanson, J R, Strickland, E M and Anson, B J (1962) Branchial sources of the auditory ossicles in man. II. Observations of embryonic stages from 7 mm to 28 mm (CR length). *Archives of Otolaryngology (Chicago)*, **76**, 200–15.

Hurst, P R, Jeffries, K, Eckstein, P and Wheeler, A G (1978) An ultrastructural study of preimplantation uterine embryos of the rhesus monkey. *Journal of Anatomy*, **126**, 209–20.

Le Dourarin, N M, Smith, J, Teillet, M-A, Le Lievre, C S and Ziller, C (1980) The neural crest and its developmental analysis in avian embryo chimaeras. *Trends in Neurosciences*, **3**, 39–42.

Luckett, W P (1978) Origin and differentiation of the yolk sac and extraembryonic mesoderm in presomite human and rhesus monkey embryos. *American Journal of Anatomy*, **152**, 59–97.

Orts-Llorca, F, Puerta Fonolla, J and Sobrado, J (1982) The formation, septation and fate of the truncus arteriosus in man. *Journal of Anatomy*, **134**, 41–56.

Pruzansky, S (1975) Roentgencephalometric studies of tonsils and adenoids in normal and pathologic states. *Annals of Otology, Rhinology and Laryngology (St Louis)*, **84**, Suppl. 19, 55–62.

Takor Takor, T and Pearse, A G E (1975) Neuroectodermal origin of avian hypothalamo-hypophyseal complex: the role of the ventral neural ridge. *Journal of Embryology and Experimental Morphology*, **34**, 311–25.

Acknowledgements

We wish to thank the following for permission to use material that has been the basis for some of the illustrations printed on the pages given in parentheses:

Edward Arnold and Co., London (page 121) from Lucas Keene, M F and Whillis, J (1950) *Anatomy for Dental Students*; Baillière, Tindall and Cox Ltd, London (page 163) from Wood Jones, F (1946) *Buchanan's Manual of Anatomy*, 7th edition; The Carnegie Institution of Washington (page 155) from Streeter, G L (1918) The developmental alterations in the vascular system of the brain of the human embryo. *Contributions to Embryology (Publications of the Carnegie Institution)*, **8**, 5–38 and (page 65) from Streeter, G L (1942, 1945, 1948) Developmental horizons in human embryos. *Contributions to Embryology (Publications of the Carnegie Institution)*, (1942) **30**, 211–245, (1945) **31**, 26–63, (1948) **32**, 133–203; J and A Churchill Ltd, London (page 165) from Ellis, R W B (1962) *Child Health and Development*, 3rd edition; W Heffer and Sons Ltd, Cambridge (pages 47, 63, 79, 145, 159) from Hamilton, W J, Boyd, J D and Mossman, H W (1962) *Human Embryology*, 3rd edition; *Journal of Anatomy* (page 61) from Hamilton, W J and Boyd, J D (1960) Development of the human placenta in the first three months of gestation. *Journal of Anatomy*, **94**, 297–328, Plate 13; Longmans, Green and Co Ltd, London (page 89) from Davies, D V and Davies, F (1962) *Gray's Anatomy*, 33rd edition; The McGraw-Hill Book Co, New York (pages 6, 64, 68, 69, 109) from Patten, Bradley M (1953) *Human Embryology*, 2nd edition; Mr M J Mycock of Hove, Sussex, England (pages 151, 153); Sandoz Ltd, Basle, Switzerland (page 159) from Dawes, G S (1958) The course of the circulation in the newborn infant. *Triangle*, **3**, 271–277; W B Saunders Co, Philadelphia (pages 121, 157) from Arey, L B (1954) *Developmental Anatomy*, 6th edition; G D Searle and Co, Chicago (page 90) from Elias, H, Functional morphology of the liver. *Research in the Service of Medicine*, **37**; Georg Thieme Verlag, Stuttgart (page 87) from Stark, D (1955) *Embryologie*; The University of Minnesota Press, Minneapolis (page 167) from Shirley, Mary M (1933) *The first two years; a study of twenty-five babies* (also appears in Faegre, Marion L and Anderson, J E, *Child Care and Training*, 7th edition); The University Tutorial Press Ltd, Cambridge (page 29) from Grove, A J and Newell, G E (1961) *Animal Biology*, 6th edition; The Wistar Institute of Anatomy and Biology, Philadelphia 4, Pa (page 155) from Barry, A (1951) Aortic arch derivatives in human adult. *Anatomical Record*, **111**, 221–238.

Ovum – – –·

Blastocyst – ·

Actual Size

0

1

2

3

4

5

6

8

Introduction

Human development begins at *conception* with *fertilization* in which a female germ cell—an *ovum*—is penetrated by a male germ cell—a *spermatozoon*. Each brings to the union a half share of hereditary information so that the single fertilized cell or *zygote* receives the full amount of information necessary for directing the development of a new individual. At the beginning the individual consists of this one cell but by the time of birth the individual consists of some 200 thousand million cells. The one cell weighs 15 ten-millionths of a gram and the newborn child weighs some 3500 g: an increase of $2\frac{1}{3}$ thousand million times during the 38 weeks between conception and birth, the period of *gestation* or pregnancy.

Gestation may be divided into pre-embryonic, embryonic and fetal periods. The *pre-embryonic period* occupies the first $2\frac{1}{2}$ weeks after conception. During the first week the zygote divides and forms a cluster of cells—the *blastocyst*—which burrows into the lining of the mother's *uterus* or womb. During the remaining week and a half, the dividing cells become arranged into *three germ layers*, surrounded by *extraembryonic membranes*. The germ layers form a pear-shaped *embryonic disc*, while the extraembryonic membranes will form the afterbirth, including the *placenta*. The *embryonic period* occupies the next $5\frac{1}{2}$ weeks. During this time the edges of the flat embryonic disc grow round and enclose head, tail and lateral folds. The edges then converge on the *umbilicus* or navel, enclosing the gut and giving the embryo a three-dimensional form. Meanwhile the basic organs and systems of the body are established from the germ layers. Thus by 8 weeks after conception the embryo, which can then be called a *fetus*, has a remarkably human external appearance with a face, hands and feet. It is, however, only 3 centimetres long and, while it has all of the major internal organs, only the heart and circulation are functioning. The *fetal period* extends from 8 weeks until birth and thus in the case of a *full-term* pregnancy lasts 30 weeks. The main features of this period are growth, the onset of other functions and changes in proportion. Growth and changes in proportion continue after birth in the postnatal period of *infancy*, *childhood*, *puberty* and *adolescence*. Puberty ends when the individual becomes capable of producing mature germ cells and beginning the process of human development anew.

Overview

The object of biology is the understanding of living systems. Living systems or organisms are not static but exhibit change. This is seen in the rapid homoeostatic cycles of everyday physiological activity and in certain more leisurely directional processes. The slowest of these is *phylogeny*—evolution—which results in diversity of form and is usually only appreciable after many generations. More rapid is the process of *ontogeny*, which leads to the maturation of an individual organism and is the province of embryology. Ontogeny begins with reproduction, of which there are two forms—asexual and sexual.

Asexual reproduction

In some multicellular animals a part of the parent body, always more than one cell, is set aside to form a new individual. The cells set aside are general body—*somatic*—cells and have the full or *diploid* number of chromosomes which bear the full complement of hereditary information. In asexual reproduction this full number is maintained in all cell divisions.

Sexual reproduction

Gametogenesis is the production of specialized generative cells or *gametes*. During the maturation of gametes the chromosome number is reduced to the half or *haploid* number. In the male, *spermatogenesis* results in a small highly motile *spermatozoon*. In the female, *oogenesis* results in a large non-motile *ovum*. The cytoplasm of the ovum contains food reserves (yolk) and exhibits regional differences which are important in subsequent development.

Fertilization is the procedure by which the spermatozoon reaches and penetrates the ovum. It leads to a series of changes in the surface of the ovum collectively termed *activation*. The nuclear derivatives of the gametes (male and female *pronuclei*) combine and the diploid number of chromosomes is restored. The process also determines the sex of the resulting *zygote*. At the time of fertilization the ovum is atypical compared with general somatic cells in that it has a very high cytoplasmic/nuclear ratio. Parthenogenetic ova develop without fertilization.

Cleavage consists of a series of mitotic divisions preceded by synthesis of nuclear material but unaccompanied by synthesis of cytoplasm. There is thus no increase in overall size and a restoration of the normal cytoplasmic/nuclear ratio eventually occurs. Cleavage results in a collection of small adherent cells, the *blastomeres*. In many chordates the blastomeres soon become arranged in the form of a hollow sphere, the *blastula*. In eutherian mammals, including

man, a cavitated sphere with somewhat different characteristics—the *blastocyst*—is formed.

Gastrulation in amphibia entails part of the wall of the blastula sinking below the surface so that a double-walled cup—the *gastrula*—is formed. The central cavity of the cup is the primitive gut or *archenteron*, and the opening to the exterior is termed the *blastopore*. Further rearrangement of the cells of the gastrula gives rise to a third layer within the double wall. The resulting three layers are the *primary germ layers*.

Primary germ layers	
ectoderm	on the outside
mesoderm	in the middle
endoderm	on the inside

The same result is achieved in other animals in different ways. Expressed in general terms, gastrulation is a complex series of movements of cell groups leading to the establishment of the primary germ layers and bringing those parts which will form the rudiments of organs into their definitive positions.

There follows a phase of *organogenesis* in which the various organ rudiments make their appearance. This gradually merges into periods dominated by *growth* and *differentiation*—both histological and functional. At an early stage of development in amniota (reptiles, birds and mammals), certain cells derived from the zygote are segregated to form a complex system of *extraembryonic membranes*. These structures support and protect the embryo, and assist in the transport of metabolites.

Embryology itself has passed through several different phases. At the outset it was *descriptive* as structural information was amassed. As descriptive data on a number of species became available, a science of *comparative* embryology emerged. The study of embryos as living systems led to *physiological* embryology. Finally, experiments designed to throw light on the causal mechanisms of development led to *analytical* or *experimental* embryology.

For ethical reasons human embryology is of necessity descriptive. Even at the descriptive level there are many gaps, particularly in the early stages, due to difficulty in obtaining material for study. Assumptions can be made about some of the gaps on the basis of comparative studies. Without such studies, many of the structural and physiological complexities of human development would be meaningless. Experimental analysis of causal mechanisms is not practicable in the case of man, and is difficult in mammals in general. Many inferences concerning developmental mechanisms are thus made from experiments in amphibia, in birds and, more recently, in rodents.

The Cell

Living tissues, mature or embryonic, consist of *cells* and *intercellular material*. Much of embryology is concerned with changes in the construction, relative position and activities of cells. Despite these changes during the developmental life of the organism, and the *differentiation* which they entail, most cells have certain elements in common. Some of these are illustrated in the diagram which represents, in simplified form, an electron micrograph of a cell after osmium tetroxide fixation.

Cytoplasm consists of a *matrix* bounded by and also permeated by a system of *cytomembranes* and containing *membrane-bound organelles*. The matrix has some properties common to colloids (e.g. sol–gel transformations) and has well-defined electrical and mechanical properties (e.g. elasticity). Parts of the membrane system may temporarily fuse and pass material from one to another, thus forming a potentially continuous system. However, each part retains its structural and functional identity during the process.

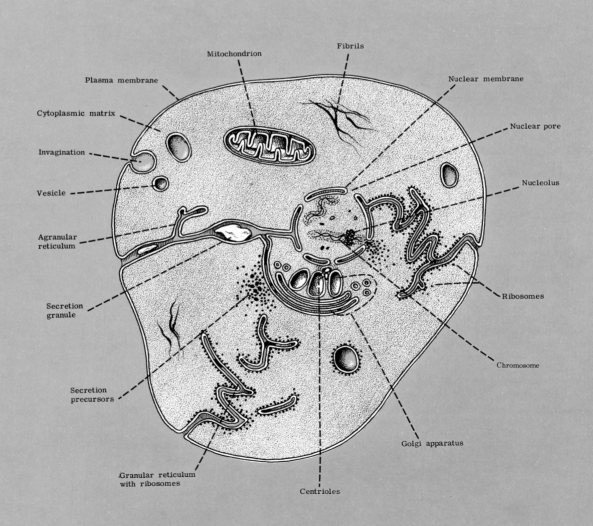

The *cytoplasm* contains *mitochondria* which are membrane-bound, usually ovoid, bodies. These are the power plants of the cell and produce substances which store the energy necessary to drive the other activities of the cell. The cytoplasm also contains sheets of membranes, collectively called *endoplasmic reticulum*, and small particles called *ribosomes*. These are the production lines of the cell which take in raw materials and manufacture substances for the maintenance of the cell itself and for the specialized activities of that cell in the body as a whole.

The *nucleus* is embedded in the cytoplasm and surrounded by its own membrane. It is the control centre and the store of hereditary information. This information is in the form of *genes* carried on *chromosomes* of which there are 46 in most human cells. Chromosomes contain *deoxyribonucleic acid* (DNA). When appropriate the genetic information is *transcribed* into a messenger substance—a type of *ribonucleic acid* (RNA)—which passes from the nucleus via pores in the nuclear membrane to convey information to the endoplasmic reticulum and ribosomes.

Before cells divide, DNA is *replicated* so that an identical set of hereditary information is available for each daughter cell. This is followed by the manufacture of other cell constituents and then by cell division. Most cell divisions are examples of *mitosis* in which the number of chromosomes is maintained and hereditary information is passed on unchanged. The production of *ova* and *spermatozoa*, however, entails *meiosis* or *reduction division* which halves the number of chromosomes and reassorts genes derived from the mother and the father. As a result, each human germ cell contains 23 chromosomes, each of which carries an admixture of maternal and paternal genes. Fertilization then results in a zygote containing 46 chromosomes—a new individual with an admixture of genes from maternal and paternal grandparents. Sex is also determined at the time of fertilization (p. 15).

During subsequent development mitotic divisions involve *proliferation* and *differentiation*—the specialization of cells. *Muscle* cells are specialized for movement and *nerve cells* for the conduction and secretion of electro-chemical signals. *Epithelial cells* cover surfaces and line cavities, being specialized for secretion and absorption. *Connective tissue cells* form the supporting elements of the body. The *basic tissues* are collections of similar specialized cells. Thus there is *muscle tissue, nerve tissue, epithelial tissue* and *connective tissue. Organs* bring the four basic tissues together in various proportions and arrangements to perform particular functions (e.g. the kidneys to excrete urine). Organs are arranged in *organ systems* which extend these functions (e.g. in the *urinary system* the *ureters* convey urine from the *kidneys* to the *bladder* which stores it until it is passed via the *urethra*). A living organism must be able to exchange material across its surfaces with the external environment, to take food, water and oxygen in and to pass waste products out. With growth in size the majority of cells have become remote from the surface and thus from direct exchange with that environment. As a result, maintaining the *internal environment* of the body becomes important and most organ systems, coupled to fluid circulatory systems, are developed to that end.

Cell structure

The highly hydrated colloidal cytoplasmic matrix or *cytosol* is bounded by the plasma and nuclear membranes, and contains numerous membrane-limited organelles (e.g. different types of vesicle, lysosomes, endoplasmic reticulum, Golgi apparatus and mitochondria). The cell therefore consists of a series of structural and functional subcellular compartments or phases of differing composition, separated from each other, or from the environment, by a variety of *cytomembranes*. These are semipermeable membranes and carry arrays of enzymatically active groups on their surfaces where many biochemical processes occur.

All membranes have two major components, *lipids* and *protein*. Individual lipid molecules are arranged as a bilayer so that their *hydrophilic* heads present to the surface and their *hydrophobic* tails are buried within the membrane. Embedded in the lipid bilayer are *integral protein* molecules which reduce its fluidity and may limit diffusion within the plane of the membrane. Given that they also act as specific enzymes and pump specific material across the membrane, the structural and functional specificity of a particular membrane depends on the content and arrangement of its proteins. The lipid of *internal cell membranes* is almost entirely *phospholipid*.

The *plasma membrane* contains *neutral lipids* and less protein than internal membranes. It has an *external coat* made up of *carbohydrate* associated with its integral protein as *glycoprotein* and its lipid as *glycolipid*. The coat, which has been shown to possess antigenic properties, 'separates' the cell from the microenvironment with which it is in constant interaction. The plasma membrane functions as a receptor surface in recognizing environmental messengers (e.g. hormones, morphogens) or other features such as the presence of foreign protein or the characteristics of neighbouring cell surfaces or of the intercellular matrix. Such information transmitted across the plasma membrane then effects alterations in the cytoplasmic machinery directly or via feedback loops. Metabolites and molecular messengers may pass 'directly' across the membrane at some point (presumably incurring a transient molecular rearrangement), may enter or leave in pinocytotic vesicles or may pass through temporary communications between the plasma membrane and other cytomembrane compartments. Some substances obey the laws of diffusion, while others are actively transported into or ejected from the cell. Active transport against concentration gradients involves expenditure of chemical energy. A good example is the preservation within the cell of a relatively high K^+ and Cl^- level and a low Na^+ level by an energy-dependent ionic pump mechanism. Such preservation of internal constancy in spite of external variations is an example of *homoeostasis* which is a fundamental attribute of living systems at all levels of organization. Finally, the plasma membrane shows well-defined mechanical and electrical properties, it partly determines cell shape and amoeboid characteristics and sometimes presents surface specializations.

The *endoplasmic reticulum* is a system of interconnecting membrane-lined channels: within the channel system secretion products are stored and transported; outside the channel system is the cytosol. The membranes contain or give attachment to many enzyme systems which are thus accessible to substrates in the cytosol; in collaboration with the Golgi complex they also elaborate new membranes, the lipid, protein and carbohydrate components being added in different regions.

Ribosomes are small particles of protein and *ribonucleic acid* (RNA) which synthesize proteins from amino acids. They occur singly or in clusters as *polysomes* which may be attached to endoplasmic reticulum. The protein synthesized by *rough* (polysome-bearing) or *granular endoplasmic reticulum* remains in membrane-bound bodies such as lyosomes or is secreted to the exterior in vesicles. The protein synthesized by unattached ribosomes or polysomes includes the enzymes and structural protein of the cytosol. *Smooth* or *agranular endoplasmic reticulum* is concerned with carbohydrate metabolism and the synthesis of lipids and steroids.

The smooth-membraned *Golgi complex* is usually located near the nucleus and consists of a series of roughly parallel flattened membranous sacs or cisternae with clusters of small vesicles near their edges. In the complex, membranes are synthesized and secretion products are modified (mainly by concentration and the addition of carbohydrate) for retention or extrusion.

Mitochondria are bounded by double membranes, the inner of which bears stalked particles and is folded into *cristae*: the cristae project into the mitochondrial *matrix*. They contain numerous enzyme systems and pumps, those of the tricarboxylic acid (Krebs') cycle being in the matrix while those of oxidative phosphorylation and the cytochrome system are carried in the inner membrane. Thus the inner membrane carries enzymes concerned with the synthesis of high-energy organic phosphate compounds, particularly *adenosine triphosphate* (ATP), which are used in energy-consuming reactions throughout the cell.

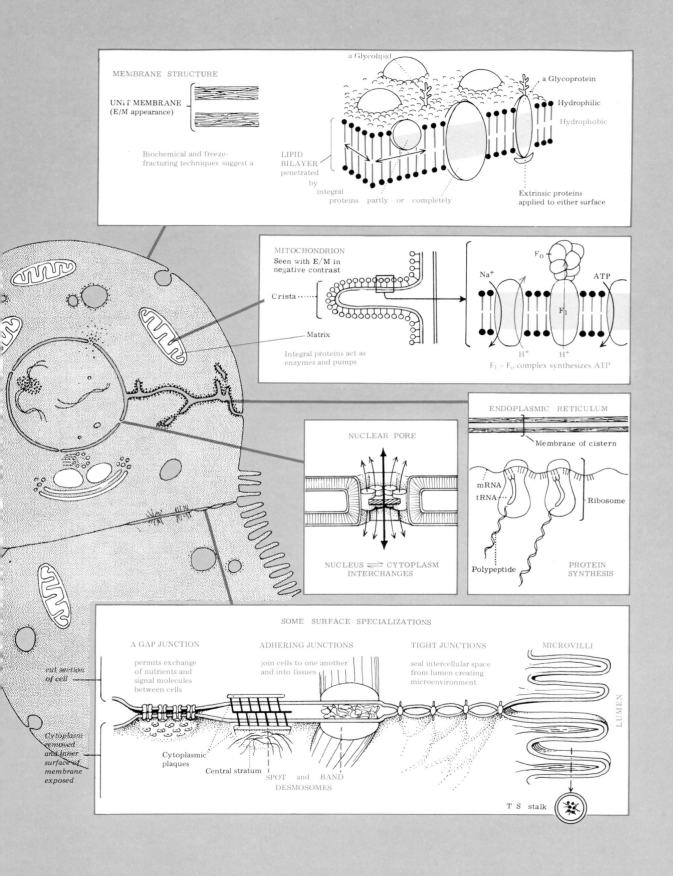

MEMBRANE STRUCTURE

UNIT MEMBRANE
(E/M appearance)

Biochemical and freeze-
fracturing techniques suggest a

a Glycolipid

a Glycoprotein

Hydrophilic

Hydrophobic

LIPID
BILAYER
penetrated
by
integral
proteins partly or completely

Extrinsic proteins
applied to either surface

MITOCHONDRION
Seen with E/M in
negative contrast

Crista

Matrix

Integral proteins act as
enzymes and pumps

F_O

Na^+

ATP

F_1

H^+ H^+

$F_1 - F_O$ complex synthesizes ATP

ENDOPLASMIC RETICULUM

Membrane of cistern

mRNA
tRNA

Ribosome

Polypeptide

PROTEIN
SYNTHESIS

NUCLEAR PORE

NUCLEUS ⇌ CYTOPLASM
INTERCHANGES

SOME SURFACE SPECIALIZATIONS

A GAP JUNCTION

permits exchange
of nutrients and
signal molecules
between cells

ADHERING JUNCTIONS

join cells to one another
and into tissues

TIGHT JUNCTIONS

seal intercellular space
from lumen creating
microenvironment

MICROVILLI

cut section
of cell

Cytoplasm
removed
and inner
surface of
membrane
exposed

Cytoplasmic
plaques

Central stratum

SPOT and BAND
DESMOSOMES

LUMEN

T S stalk

Organelles and replication

Lysosomes are a heterogeneous group of membrane-bound organelles containing a dense matrix which is rich in hydrolytic enzymes. They are associated with the intracellular breakdown of ingested particles or with cellular turnover, degeneration and tissue remodelling.

The *centrioles* are a pair of minute cylindrical bodies set at right angles to each other. In cross-section each cylinder presents a spiralized ring of nine triple tubules. They are concerned with the synthesis of microtubules, including those of the achromatic spindle which is a feature of the dividing cell.

The *nuclear membrane* is double: the outer membrane is often continuous externally with other cytomembranes, usually the granular endoplasmic reticulum. The two membranes become continuous at the margins of the fine nuclear 'pores' which are the sites of nucleocytoplasmic interchange of large molecules (e.g. RNA and various proteins). Electrical impedance studies show that in some cells the pores are not always 'patent'.

The *nuclear matrix* contains the chromosomes and one or more nucleoli. A *nucleolus* is an RNA-rich organelle, organized on the nucleolar zones of particular chromosomes, and concerned with the synthesis of ribosomal RNA.

Chromosomes consist of a linear array of *deoxyribonucleic acid* (DNA) molecules associated with various proteins and small amounts of RNA and bearing coded hereditary information. DNA and RNA are polynucleotides (nucleotide = base-sugar-phosphate) and have a spirally disposed backbone, in which sugar and phosphate groups alternate, with bases projecting laterally from the sugar towards the axis of the spiral. In DNA the sugar is deoxyribose and the bases are the purines, adenine (A) and guanine (G), and the pyrimidines, thymine (T) and cytosine (C). The macromolecule of DNA consists of an extremely long, complementary pair of helices linked through their base side chains in such a way that A always links with T and G with C. As a prelude to cell division the nuclear DNA exhibits one of its most characteristic properties—synthesis involving replication of its macromolecular structure. *Replication* is the means by which the daughter cells which result from cell division can receive macromolecules of DNA which bear a sequence of bases identical with that of the parent cell. It is the sequence of base pairs in the DNA which conveys the information that ultimately directs the sequential addition of amino acids during protein synthesis. Each triplet (group of three base pairs) forms a code unit which specifies which single amino acid is to be added. Replication occurs during the S (*synthetic*) period of the cell cycle and takes about 7 hours. The manufacture of proteins to be used in cell division takes place in the succeeding G2 (*second gap*) period of up to 5 hours. Chromosomes are segregated in the M (*mitosis*) period and the parent cell separates into two in the D (*division*) period. Mitotic division takes about 1 hour and is succeeded by a G1 (*first gap*) resting period which may last from a few hours to many years. G1 and G2 are considerably foreshortened in cleavage in early development.

In the phase between cell divisions, varying parts of the chromosomes are condensed and stain as *heterochromatin*. Other parts are dispersed and do not stain readily—*euchromatin*. The regions which are euchromatic at a particular time are actively engaged in *transcription*, the initial stage of protein synthesis. In this process the base sequence of one of the DNA helices is transcribed into the complementary base sequence of a long-chain, single helix of a *messenger* polynucleotide (mRNA) in the nucleus. In *RNA* (compared with DNA) the sugar is ribose (instead of deoxyribose) and one of the bases is uracil (instead of thymine). The strip of mRNA, bearing the code, is transported to the cytoplasm via nuclear pores. Here it associates with the structural, non-informative, RNA of ribosomes. Each ribosome attaches to one end of the messenger and travels along its length, eventually to detach at the other end. The amino acids free within the cytoplasm become *activated* and join a short double-helix of soluble (or *transfer*) tRNA. A specific tRNA exists for each amino acid. As the ribosome proceeds along the messenger strip, the base triplet code carried by the messenger is 'read' by the active end groups of the tRNA. Only one of the active end groups will fit at each code triplet. In this manner the polypeptide chain grows in length as each amino acid is added in a sequence originally determined by the ultrastructure of the nuclear DNA.

Nucleic Acids

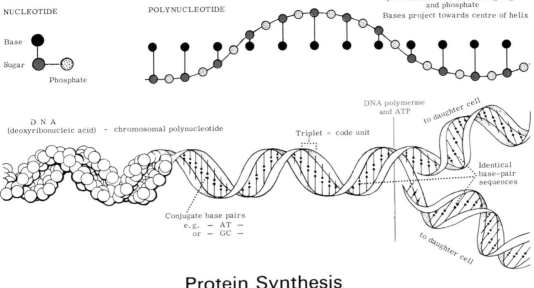

NUCLEOTIDE

Base

Sugar

Phosphate

POLYNUCLEOTIDE

Spiral backbone of alternating sugar and phosphate

Bases project towards centre of helix

D N A
(deoxyribonucleic acid) - chromosomal polynucleotide

Triplet = code unit

DNA polymerase and ATP

to daughter cell

Identical base-pair sequences

Conjugate base pairs
e.g. — AT —
or — GC —

to daughter cell

Protein Synthesis

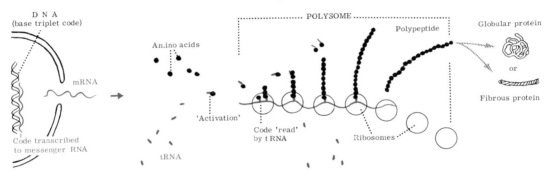

D N A
(base triplet code)

mRNA

Code transcribed to messenger RNA

Amino acids

'Activation'

tRNA

POLYSOME

Polypeptide

Code 'read' by t RNA

Ribosomes

Globular protein

or

Fibrous protein

Interphase Chromosomes and Cell Cycle

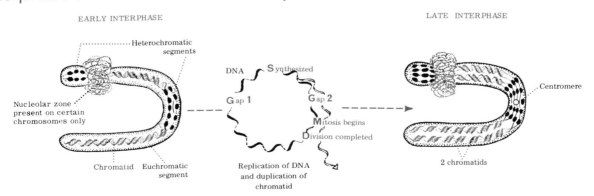

EARLY INTERPHASE

LATE INTERPHASE

Heterochromatic segments

Nucleolar zone present on certain chromosomes only

Chromatid Euchromatic segment

DNA Synthesized

Gap 1 Gap 2

Mitosis begins

Division completed

Replication of DNA and duplication of chromatid

Centromere

2 chromatids

13

Control of Gene Action

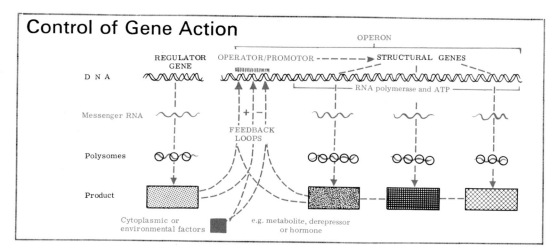

That part of the DNA molecule which specifies a single polypeptide chain is termed a *structural gene* and has a short initiating segment of *operator/promotor*. Where a protein consists of a number of chains the common operator/promotor and its associated structural genes are termed an *operon*. Other regions operate as *regulator genes* and enhance (*derepress*) or diminish (*repress*) the activity of neighbouring operons. It is thought that regulator gene product reacts with a cytoplasmic or environmental factor and that this combined product completes a feedback loop by controlling the structural gene through its operator.

Most operons are kept inactive (*blocked*) by the action of non-specific basic nucleoproteins (*histones*) on the operator. A non-histone acid protein which is specific for a particular operon *deblocks* it by disengaging its histones from the operator, permitting the binding of RNA polymerases to the promotor and initiating transcription in the structural genes. Each cell of the body carries an identical complement of genes—the *genome*—but in each different type of cell the genome is expressed differently because the greater part of it is kept blocked and not used. The level of activity of a particular cell depends on the

extent to which its unblocked genes are derepressed.

Although separate chromosomes are indistinguishable between cell divisions they retain their individuality. In the S period of a cell cycle they replicate so that each chromosome entering prophase consists of two identical *chromatids*. As cell division progresses the chromosomes coil on themselves, condense and become demonstrable by light microscopy. The stages of mitotic division may then be followed. The essential feature of *mitosis* is that the diploid number of chromosomes and the genetic constitution of the cell are perpetuated.

When whole chromosomes become demonstrable in mitosis the total complement may be studied. In normal human somatic cells there are 46 chromosomes. This is known as the diploid number (2n = 46) since the haploid number (n = 23) was received from each parent at the time of fertilization. The diploid set may thus be arranged as a series of 23 pairs of homologous chromosomes, one member of each pair being of maternal origin and one of paternal origin. As a corollary the chromosome number must be reduced from diploid to haploid during the formation of ova and sperms in gametogenesis.

Mitosis   DIPLOID NUMBER OF CHROMOSOMES AND GENETIC CONSTITUTION PERPETUATED

INTERPHASE	PROPHASE	METAPHASE	ANAPHASE	TELOPHASE
Replication of DNA and duplication of chromatid	Cell rounds up, nucleolus and nuclear membrane disappear. Centrioles move to opposite poles and an achromatic spindle forms. Chromosomes (each consisting of two chromatids) become stainable	Centromeres 'attach' to equator of spindle	Centromeres divide into two parts each with an associated chromatid. These parts separate and take their chromatids to opposite poles of the spindle	Cytoplasmic division and nuclear reconstitution in the two daughter cells

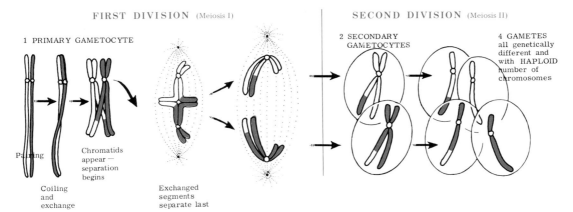

FIRST DIVISION (Meiosis I)

1 PRIMARY GAMETOCYTE

Pairing

Coiling
and
exchange

Chromatids
appear—
separation
begins

Exchanged
segments
separate last

SECOND DIVISION (Meiosis II)

2 SECONDARY
GAMETOCYTES

4 GAMETES
all genetically
different and
with HAPLOID
number of
chromosomes

The somatic cells of an organism are conventionally regarded as being genetically identical and mitotic divisions as conserving this genetic identity. *Gametogenesis*, however, entails meiotic divisions which result in the segregation and redistribution of genetic material. Early in gametogenesis, DNA is replicated, chromatids are duplicated (but remain latent) and *meiosis (reduction division)* begins with the pairing of homologous chromosomes. The fate of a single pair may be followed in the diagram. During coiling, segments of DNA—genetic material—are exchanged between chromosomes. After shortening, the two chromatids of each chromosome are revealed and separation begins as their centromeres move to opposite poles. Exchanged segments are the last to separate. More than one exchange may occur in a single chromosome pair. This first division—*meiosis I*—reduces the chromosome number by one-half to the haploid number, but, because DNA was replicated and the chromatids duplicated beforehand, each of the chromosomes of a secondary gametocyte consists of two chromatids.

At the second division—*meiosis II*—these chromatids separate and become the chromosomes of four gametes. From the original homologous pair of chromosomes four haploid gametes have been pro-

duced—each with a different set of chromosomes and genes. Where, as in man, a number of homologous pairs of chromosomes are present at the onset of meiosis, the gene content of a particular gamete will depend on the number of exchanges between maternal and paternal chromosomes, the possible combinations being innumerable. The resulting redistribution of genetic material, together with those as yet causally unexplained genetic changes called *mutations*, produces diversity of form in the offspring. It is on such variations that the forces of natural selection operate and effect evolutionary change.

Of the total complement of 46 chromosomes, 44 are not concerned in sex determination and are called *autosomes*. The remaining pair determine the sex of the individual and are called *sex chromosomes*. In the female the pair are similar and are called X chromosomes. In the male only one is an X chromosome. The other, which is called the Y chromosome, is much smaller and bears genes the products of which are actively male-determining. By convention the total number of chromosomes is written first, then the sex chromosomes, then any anomaly. Thus the normal female and male are written as 46,XX and 46,XY respectively.

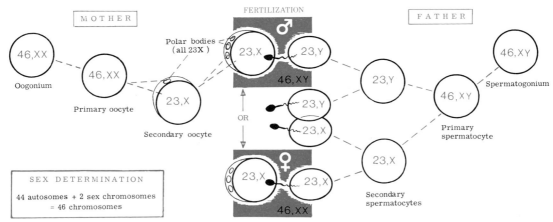

FERTILIZATION

MOTHER

FATHER

46,XX

Oogonium

46,XX

Primary oocyte

23,X

Secondary oocyte

Polar bodies
(all 23X)

♂

23,X   23,Y

46,XY

23,Y

23,X

OR

♀

23,X   23,X

46,XX

23,Y

23,X

Secondary
spermatocytes

46,XY

Primary
spermatocyte

46,XY

Spermatogonium

SEX DETERMINATION

44 autosomes + 2 sex chromosomes
= 46 chromosomes

15

Cytogenetics

One X chromosome being necessary and sufficient for normal development, only one of the X chromosomes in a female cell (randomly determined for each cell line) is active. The other remains relatively inactive and heterochromatic, and appears as a dark-staining body (*Barr body* or *sex chromatin*) beneath the nuclear membrane. The normal female is said to be chromatin-positive. By examination of, for example, cells scraped from the inside of the cheek, the number of X chromosomes may be inferred. There is always one more than the number of Barr bodies.

When cells in metaphase are examined in squash preparations, the chromosomal constitution or *karyotype* may be determined by arranging the chromosomes in pairs, in descending order of length and according to the position of the centromere. The centromere which is the site of linkage between the two chromatids may be approximately at the centre of its length (*metacentric*), near its end (*acrocentric*) or in between (*submetacentric*). Identification of individual chromosomes is facilitated by the staining of characteristic horizontal bands.

Abnormal cell division

Cell division does not always proceed harmoniously and nearly 1 zygote in 10 has an identifiable chromosomal anomaly. The commonest source is non-disjunction, the failure of one or more homologous pairs of chromosomes or chromatids to separate during cell division. If non-disjunction occurs in meiosis, some gametes receive both and others neither of the homologous chromosomes. Fusion with a haploid gamete from the other parent then results in a zygote with three (*trisomy*) or only one (*monosomy*) of the chromosome concerned and one more (47) or one less (45) than the normal diploid number in total. If the whole set fail to separate, multiples of the haploid number (e.g. *triploidy*, *tetraploidy*, etc.) result. *Mosaicism* is the presence in an individual of two or more cell lines. In a sense all females are mosaics because some cells carry an active maternal X chromosome and others an active paternal X chromosome. Cell lines with different karyotypes may result from non-disjunction in a mitotic division in early embryonic life.

The more genetic imbalance that results from an anomaly, the more likely is the gamete to be non-viable or the conceptus to be rejected as a spontaneous abortion; less severe imbalance results in live birth of abnormal individuals. Thus monosomies of the autosomes and trisomies of the large autosomes are not seen even in abortuses. There the commonest anomalies are triploidy (69), trisomy 16 (47, +16) and monosomy X (45,X or XO). Triploidy and trisomy 16 are not seen in live-born children, except in mosaics, but some XO genotypes, perhaps 1 in 20, survive and

the *genotype* is expressed as the *phenotype* known as Turner's syndrome (*ovarian dysgenesis*).

Among live-born children, trisomy 21 (47, +21) and trisomy X (47,XXX or 47,XXY) are the commonest anomalies. About half of the trisomy 21 genotypes abort; the remainder become cases of Down's syndrome (*mongolism*). Few of the trisomy X genotypes abort, the excess X chromosomes remaining relatively inactive and forming additional Barr bodies. The excess chromosomes do, however, have some effect on fertility and intelligence which may be impaired in the phenotypes associated with XXX (female) and XXY (male with Klinefelter's syndrome). The XYY genotype is probably as common but is less frequently diagnosed as the individual may be phenotypically normal. Polysomy X and trisomies 13 and 18 also occur but the trisomies rarely survive infancy.

Other anomalies arise from chromosomal breaks. Breaks in chromatids during exchange are normal; other breaks are not uncommon but normally unite without anomaly. However, segments between or beyond breaks may be lost (*deletion*) or fuse with another non-homologous chromosome (*translocation*). Deletion of material from the X chromosome makes a female monosomic for that material and results in ovarian dysgenesis with 46 chromosomes and a single small Barr body. A translocation which occurs during mitosis is balanced since the total complement of genetic material—the genome—is unchanged and the individual is phenotypically normal. In gametogenesis, however, the translocated chromosome will pair with one of its source chromosomes so that some gametes will have an excess and others a deficiency of the genetic material normally carried on the other source chromosome. Thus a parent with a fusion chromosome in which some 21 material is attached to 15 will have only 45 chromosomes but be phenotypically normal. Some of the offspring, however, will receive the fusion chromosome plus a 21 chromosome from each parent, will thus be trisomic for 21 and will present as Down's syndrome with 46 chromosomes. Finally, a transverse instead of a longitudinal break at the centromere results in two abnormal *isochromosomes*: a small one made up of two sets of short-arm material and a large one made up of two sets of long-arm material. An individual with an isochromosome and a normal homologous chromosome will have an excess (trisomy) of genetic material normally carried on one arm and a deficiency (monosomy) of material normally carried on the other. Thus an isochromosome of the long arm of chromosome 21 makes an individual trisomic for it and again results in Down's syndrome with 46 chromosomes; an isochromosome of the long arm of the X chromosome makes a female monosomic for short-arm material and results in ovarian dysgenesis with 46 chromosomes and a single large Barr body.

Human Chromosomes

Diagrammatic representation (Ideogram) of the
NORMAL MALE CHROMOSOME COMPLEMENT (46,XY)

Group A (1 − 3)   are large and metacentric

Group B (4 − 5)   are large and submetacentric

Group C (6 − 12 and X) are medium sized and
                  submetacentric

Group D (13 − 15) are medium sized and acrocentric
                  with satellites on the short arms

Group E (16 − 18) are rather short and metacentric
                  or submetacentric

Group F (19 − 20) are short and metacentric

Group G (21 − 22 and Y) are very short and acro-
        centric, 21 and 22 having satellites.

*RED is used on this page
to denote abnormalities*

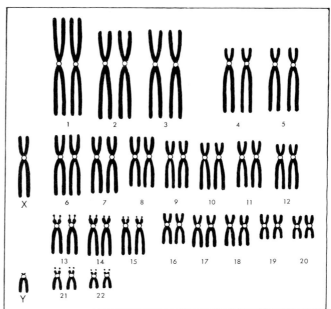

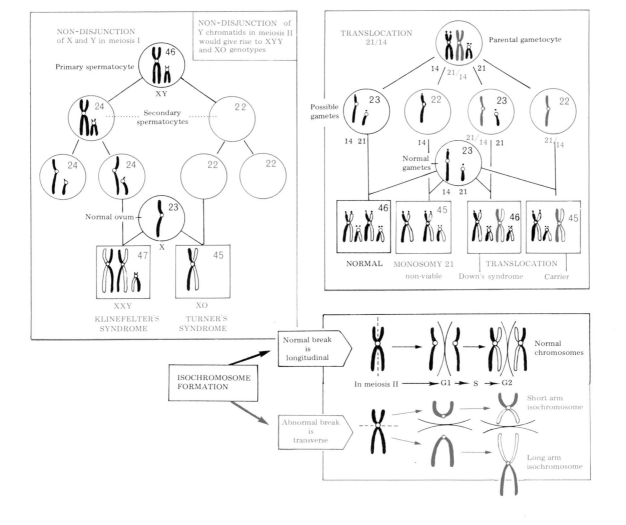

Autosomal inheritance

The site at which a gene is found on a chromosome is called a *gene locus* and the alternative genes which can occupy that site are called *alleles*. For example, at the locus concerned with the production of substances which determine the ABO blood group the alleles are the A genes (A_1 and A_2), a B gene and an O gene. The A and B alleles (but not the O allele) are responsible for the conversion of substrate H into their identifiable *gene products*, the A and B red cell antigens respectively. There are corresponding gene loci on each of the autosomes in a homologous pair so that any individual has two ABO alleles, the possible genotypes being A/A, A/O, B/B, B/O, A/B and O/O. In these genotypes one of the alleles will be derived from each of the individual's parents because *alleles segregate* in gametogenesis and pass into different haploid gametes (*Mendel's first law*), permitting new combinations in the offspring.

The genotypes A/A, B/B and O/O having matching alleles at the two homologous gene loci are said to be *homozygous*. The genotypes A/O, B/O and A/B, having unlike alleles at the two loci, are said to be *heterozygous*. If either A or B or both are present, H is converted and the genotype is expressed in the phenotype of the individual. Thus both the homozygote A/A and the heterozygote A/O produce A antigens and they both present with the phenotype blood group A. Only the homozygote O/O fails to convert H which is thus found in the red cells of phenotype group O. Genes which are expressed in the phenotypes of heterozygotes are said to be *dominant*, whilst those which are expressed only in the homozygote are said to be *recessive*; A and B are dominant and O is recessive. Just as normal alleles show dominance and recessiveness so do disease-producing mutant alleles, in all some 2000 conditions having been described.

In conditions showing *autosomal dominant inheritance* the first affected person in a family is so as a result of a fresh mutation in one gene of the homologous pair. The person is thus heterozygous and produces gametes bearing the normal and mutant alleles in equal numbers. An unaffected mate produces only gametes bearing the normal allele so that there is a 1 in 2 chance of a child being affected regardless of its sex. The other characteristics of autosomal dominant inheritance are that every generation is affected and that only the affected transmit the condition. Severe dominant diseases continue in the population as a result of fresh mutations but tend to breed themselves out of families. This may not happen if the onset of the condition occurs late in reproductive life as in Huntington's chorea or if as is commonly the case there is variation in the extent to which the mutant gene is expressed in the phenotype.

In conditions showing *autosomal recessive inheritance* the first affected person in a family is so as a result of receiving a mutant allele from each of the parents who are heterozygous carriers of the condition. Such is more likely to be the case in first-cousin or other consanguineous matings. The parents produce gametes bearing normal and mutant alleles in equal numbers and the chances of a child being affected (or of a second child being affected) are 1 in 4 regardless of its sex. In some instances heterozygous carriers may be detected by enzyme assays; their incidence in a population may be inferred from the Hardy–Weinberg equation and proves to be surprisingly high.

According to the Hardy–Weinberg law, if there are two or more alleles in a population then, in the absence of selection or selective mating, their proportions remain the same from generation to generation. For two alleles this may be expressed as $p^2 + 2pq + q^2 = 1$, where p and q are the frequencies of the alleles, p^2 and q^2 those of the homozygotes and $2pq$ that of the heterozygote. The commonest autosomal recessive disease is *cystic fibrosis*, a condition in which the pancreatic, bronchial and other exocrine secretions are abnormal. It has an incidence (p^2) of 1 in 2000 births. Thus the frequency of the mutant allele (p) is

$$\sqrt{1/2000} = 0.02$$

the frequency of the normal allele (q) is

$$1 - 0.02 = 0.98$$

and the frequency of the heterozygote ($2pq$) is therefore

$$2 \times 0.02 \times 0.98 = 0.04, \text{ or } 1 \text{ in } 25.$$

GAMETOGENESIS and ABO BLOOD GROUPS

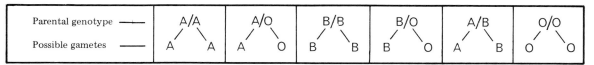

Parental genotype ——	A/A	A/O	B/B	B/O	A/B	O/O
Possible gametes ——	A A	A O	B B	B O	A B	O O

MENDEL'S FIRST LAW — alleles segregate in gametogenesis

BLOOD GROUP TYPES

Genotype	A/A	A/O	B/B	B/O	A/B	O/O
Zygosity	Homozygous	Heterozygous	Homozygous	Heterozygous	Heterozygous	Homozygous
Antigen (gene product)	A	A	B	B	A + B	H
Phenotype (blood group)	A		B		AB	O

Genes are expressed in the phenotype by their gene product

AUTOSOMAL DOMINANT INHERITANCE

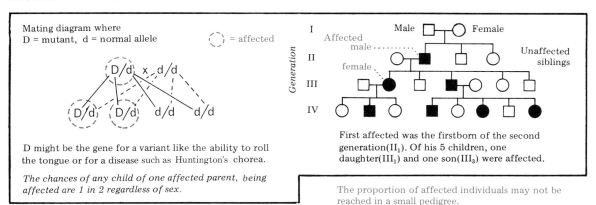

Mating diagram where D = mutant, d = normal allele

( ) = affected

D might be the gene for a variant like the ability to roll the tongue or for a disease such as Huntington's chorea.

The chances of any child of one affected parent, being affected are 1 in 2 regardless of sex.

First affected was the firstborn of the second generation(II$_1$). Of his 5 children, one daughter(III$_1$) and one son(III$_3$) were affected.

The proportion of affected individuals may not be reached in a small pedigree.

AUTOSOMAL RECESSIVE INHERITANCE

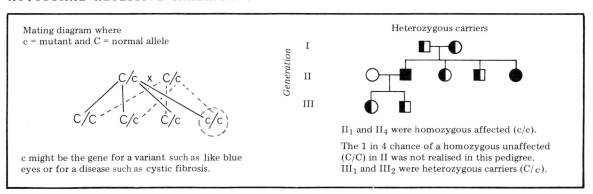

Mating diagram where c = mutant and C = normal allele

Heterozygous carriers

c might be the gene for a variant such as like blue eyes or for a disease such as cystic fibrosis.

II$_1$ and II$_4$ were homozygous affected (c/c).

The 1 in 4 chance of a homozygous unaffected (C/C) in II was not realised in this pedigree. III$_1$ and III$_2$ were heterozygous carriers (C/c).

The chances of any child of heterozygous parents, being affected are 1 in 4 regardless of sex.

Linked and polygenic inheritance

The inheritance of a gene on the X chromosome is described as *X-linked*. Such a gene is always expressed in the male because there is no corresponding alternative gene to be expressed on the Y chromosome; in the female, however, it may be expressed only in the homozygote (recessive) or, more rarely, also in the heterozygote (dominant). In *X-linked recessive inheritance*, the first affected person in a family is usually a male who has received a mutant allele from his heterozygous mother. Since she produces gametes bearing normal and mutant alleles in equal numbers the chances of a son being affected and of a daughter being a heterozygous carrier are both 1 in 2. Males are affected much more often than females and transmit the condition through all their daughters to half of their sons. In *X-linked dominant inheritance*, the daughters of an affected male are all affected while the chances of the children of a heterozygous woman being affected are 1 in 2 regardless of sex. The Y chromosome probably has no genes on it apart from those directly or indirectly determining masculinity; no Y-linked diseases are known.

Linkage has a further connotation. Whereas alleles segregate and pass into different gametes, non-alleles (members of different gene pairs) may pass into the same or different gametes. If the loci concerned are on different chromosomes or far apart on the same chromosome, *non-alleles assort* independently (*Mendel's second law*); when they are close together on the same chromosome, non-alleles pass into different gametes with a frequency of less than 50 per cent and are said to be linked. Linked genes are less likely to be separated in the exchange of material between homologous chromosomes which occurs only in gametogenesis. Thus for a given pair of non-alleles the percentage of recombinant genotypes (differing from those of either parent) is a measure of the distance apart of their loci and can be used to plot genes on chromosomes.

Genetic linkage is to be distinguished from *association*, which is the non-random occurrence of two genetically separate traits in a population. For example, blood group O and duodenal ulcer show significant *association*, but, because they are not attributable to genes on the same chromosome, *linkage* is not involved.

It was originally thought that the ABO blood groups were determined by two non-alleles A and B.

However, the fact that the progeny of an AB × O mating is always A or B and never AB or O shows that A and B always segregate and are thus alleles; the phenotype frequencies also agree with those predicted by the Hardy–Weinberg law for a multiple allele system.

Polymorphism

Segregation, independent and linked assortment and mutations are the sources of *genetic polymorphism*— 'The occurrence together in the same habitat of two or more discontinuous forms of a species in such proportions that the rarest of them cannot be maintained merely by recurrent mutation' (E. B. Ford). If a mutant gene is wholly disadvantageous (which it usually is) or wholly advantageous, the polymorphism is transient as the mutant is either bred out or takes over from the normal allele respectively. For *balanced polymorphism* the mutant must be neutral (which it rarely is) or confer a selective advantage in some situations to compensate for others. While many polymorphic systems exist, few of these selective factors are known. The normal and sickle-cell haemoglobin system (Hb-A and Hb^S) is an exception. About 1 in 25 newborn children in some East African populations are homozygous for the mutant (Hb^S/Hb^S) and have sickle-cell anaemia from which most of them die in infancy. Yet 1 in 25 homozygotes (p^2) means a mutant gene frequency (p) of 1 in 5. The reason for this high frequency is that the young heterozygotes (Hb^A/Hb^S) are more resistant to malignant malaria and have this selective advantage over the normal homozygote (Hb^A/Hb^A). In the ABO blood group system genetic predisposition to particular diseases may be the selective factor.

The foregoing considerations apply where the character studied is either the gene product or a distinct feature related to it. There are, however, other characteristics such as height and blood pressure which are measured rather than counted and are distributed continuously rather than bimodally. These characteristics and many disease conditions depend upon genetic variation at more than one gene locus with no individual gene making a predominant contribution to the variation; this is *polygenic inheritance*. The total determination of the character or condition, however, depends not only on genetic but also on environmental factors which together affect how genes are expressed in the phenotype; this is *multifactorial inheritance*.

X-LINKED RECESSIVE INHERITANCE

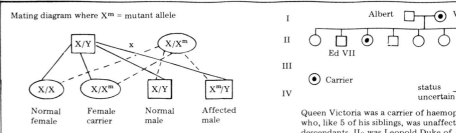

Mating diagram where X^m = mutant allele

The chances of a male child of a female carrier being affected are 1 in 2 as are those of a female child being a carrier.

Ed VII

Carrier

status uncertain →

Queen Victoria was a carrier of haemophilia. II_2 was Edward VII who, like 5 of his siblings, was unaffected and had no affected descendants. II_8 was Leopold Duke of Albany who died of haemophilia. He had a carrier daughter III_1 and she and her aunts II_3 and II_9 had haemophiliac sons.

X-LINKED DOMINANT INHERITANCE

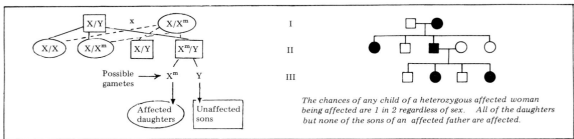

Possible gametes

Affected daughters

Unaffected sons

The chances of any child of a heterozygous affected woman being affected are 1 in 2 regardless of sex. All of the daughters but none of the sons of an affected father are affected.

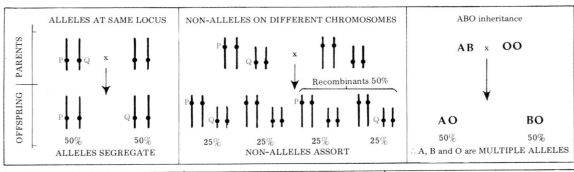

PARENTS

OFFSPRING

ALLELES AT SAME LOCUS

50%   50%

ALLELES SEGREGATE

NON-ALLELES ON DIFFERENT CHROMOSOMES

Recombinants 50%

25%   25%   25%   25%

NON-ALLELES ASSORT

ABO inheritance

AB x OO

AO   BO

50%   50%

∴ A, B and O are MULTIPLE ALLELES

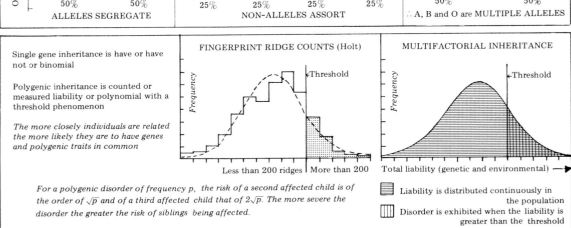

Single gene inheritance is have or have not or binomial

Polygenic inheritance is counted or measured liability or polynomial with a threshold phenomenon

The more closely individuals are related the more likely they are to have genes and polygenic traits in common

FINGERPRINT RIDGE COUNTS (Holt)

Frequency

Threshold

Less than 200 ridges | More than 200

MULTIFACTORIAL INHERITANCE

Frequency

Threshold

Total liability (genetic and environmental) →

For a polygenic disorder of frequency p, the risk of a second affected child is of the order of $\sqrt{p}$ and of a third affected child that of $2\sqrt{p}$. The more severe the disorder the greater the risk of siblings being affected.

Liability is distributed continuously in the population

Disorder is exhibited when the liability is greater than the threshold

Growth

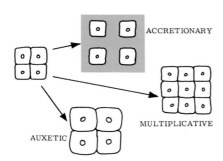

ACCRETIONARY

MULTIPLICATIVE

AUXETIC

Cell Cycles

Cell cycles may be proliferative or quantal

Most genes are blocked and inactive and remain so in proliferative cycles.

In quantal cycles some genes are deblocked, others reblocked and a different cell line results.

PROLIFERATIVE

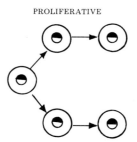

A precise definition of *growth* is difficult, but a useful approximation is—*the increase in weight or size of all or part of an organism which follows the synthesis of protoplasm, or of those extracellular products that are integral parts of the tissues of the organism.* Simple ingestion of material does not constitute growth. Growth of a cellular aggregate may be *accretionary* (due to an increase in intercellular material), *multiplicative* (due to an increase in number of cells) or *auxetic* (due to an increase in size of the cells). In practice, programmed combinations of these types of growth are balanced by programmed regression, degeneration and cell death to produce differential growth patterns. Cell division may be inhibited by secretions of the aggregate itself, called *chalones*.

Mitotic cell cycles may be *proliferative* (resulting in growth) or *quantal* (resulting in different daughter cells by the deblocking of different parts of the genome). By means of sequential quantal cycles a

primitive cell is potentially able to specialize along many different lines—in this sense it is pluripotent. However, each quantal cycle is a point at which a cell is bipotential and its daughter cells may enter one of two paths. Quantal cycles thus result in *differentiation—the acquisition of phenotypic variation amongst cells of identical genotype*. When quantal cycles occur depends upon interplay between genetic, cytoplasmic and environmental factors.

When a cell with regional differences in its cytoplasm divides it gives rise to daughter cells with different nucleocytoplasmic relationships. Different cytoplasmic feedback loops and different gene combinations then become operative, and the cells may develop along different lines. Alternatively, two daughter cells, initially similar, may become exposed to different microenvironments. Again, different feedback loops and gene combinations may become operative. The microenvironment of a cell depends

PROGRESSIVE RESTRICTION OF POSSIBLE FATES AND ESTABLISHMENT OF CELL LINES

CHEMO-DIFFERENTIATION (determination)

CYTO-DIFFERENTIATION

HISTO-DIFFERENTIATION

FUNCTIONAL DIFFERENTIATION

'Undifferentiated' cell

| GENETIC FACTORS | | CYTOPLASMIC FACTORS | | ENVIRONMENTAL FACTORS e.g. metabolites, hormones, derepressors etc. |

Differentiation

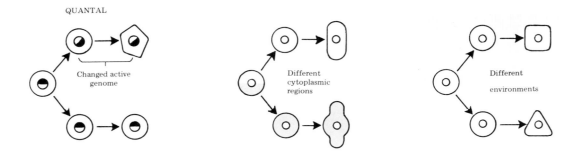

QUANTAL

Changed active genome

Different cytoplasmic regions

Different environments

upon its position in an aggregate, its contacts with neighbouring cells and matrix, and the presence of chemical messengers (hormones, derepressors, etc.). The effects of a conditioning environment may be permanent and may restrict the possible fates of a cell and its descendants (*differentiation*), or be temporary and persist only as long as the conditioning environment is present (*modulation*).

The fate of a cell is *determined* (*chemodifferentiation*) before visible changes occur. Observable cytological changes (*cytodifferentiation*) are followed by the welding of various types into a structurally organized tissue (*histodifferentiation*). Full differentiation is achieved with the onset of function in a tissue.

Pattern formation is the process whereby apparently similar members of an aggregate of cells differentiate along different paths in an ordered sequence in space and time. Whether the immediate source of pattern is to be sought in the genome or in intercellular communication via antigens or via gap junctions which are present from the 8-cell stage is a matter of conjecture. Regardless of their source, patterns which entail polarity, axes and gradients are present throughout development.

Until a few years ago most of the experiments on

the mechanisms of vertebrate development were carried out on amphibia. At the end of cleavage the *amphibian blastula* consists of a hollow sphere of cells enclosing a cavity—the *blastocoele*. At the *animal pole* the cells are small and pigmented; at the *vegetative pole* they are large, pale and laden with yolk. If small regions of the blastula are stained with a vital dye, their fate in subsequent development may be followed. It is thus possible to say, for instance, that the cells of the animal pole normally give rise to ectoderm. From the results of many such experiments, maps indicating *presumptive fate* may be drawn. More recently, the production of *composite blastocysts* by the transplanting of identifiable rat cells into mouse blastocoeles has permitted the production of similar maps for a mammal.

Morphogenesis is the attainment of the appropriate spatial and temporal relationships between phenotypically distinct cells. This process, entailing as it does differential growth and movement, is dramatically exemplified by *gastrulation*, which leads to the establishment of the primary germ layers and brings presumptive organ rudiments into their definitive positions.

Gastrulation

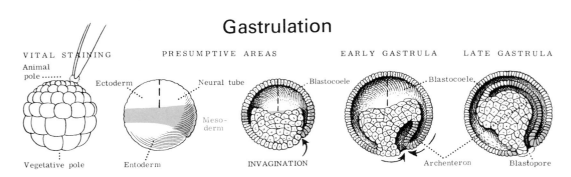

VITAL STAINING

Animal pole

Vegetative pole

PRESUMPTIVE AREAS

Ectoderm

Neural tube

Meso-derm

Entoderm

EARLY GASTRULA

Blastocoele

INVAGINATION

LATE GASTRULA

Blastocoele

Archenteron

Blastopore

Developmental Mechanisms

In amphibia *gastrulation* entails spreading of the animal pole cells over the vegetative cells so that the *presumptive endoderm* and *chorda-mesoderm* become invaginated. This results in obliteration of the blastocoele and the formation of another cavity—the primitive gut or *archenteron*. The archenteron communicates with the exterior through the *blastopore*. The roof of the archenteron consists of the chorda-mesoderm which now lies in contact with the overlying *presumptive neural tube*. The further development of the nervous system is dependent on influences originating in the chorda-mesoderm and affecting the overlying presumptive tissue. For example, a piece of presumptive neural tube taken before gastrulation and cultured in a salt solution formed a sheet of epithelium. What it would have become depended on *where* it was, not *what* it was—it had not been *determined* as neural tissue. When a similar piece was taken from a late gastrula it differentiated into neural tissue. What it became depended on *what* it was—it had been *determined* as neural tissue.

The region of the blastopore through which invagination of chorda-mesoderm takes place is its dorsal lip. General body mesoderm proliferates from the lateral lips of the blastopore which approach each other and fuse, forming the *primitive streak*. The original blastopore is thus divided by the primitive streak into dorsal and ventral orifices. Since the hind end of the neural plate borders the blastopore, the dorsal orifice will connect the cavity of the neural tube with the archenteron and form a transient *neurenteric canal*. The ventral orifice connects the archenteron with the exterior and forms the future *cloaca*.

Removal of the dorsal lip of the blastopore from an early gastrula prevents further development. On the other hand, transplantation of the dorsal lip from one early gastrula into an undetermined region of another, induces the formation of a second embryonic axis. This depends upon the presence of the dorsal lip derivative—chorda-mesoderm. The establishment of the embryonic axis depends upon the neuralizing and mesodermalizing effects of the chorda-mesoderm on the overlying presumptive neural tissue. The *neuralizing* effect alone induces forebrain and associated structures whereas the *mesodermalizing* effect alone induces such structures as notochord, somites and kidneys. The *induction* of an organized nervous system with correct orientation of its parts is due to the graded interaction of these two effects. Quite how the process works is not known; in some cases, but by no means all, intimate cell-to-cell contacts appear necessary for induction and the effect is spread by cell *migration*.

Other interactions between cell surfaces are also important in morphogenesis: *contact guidance* describes the way certain cells move along preferred pathways; *contact inhibition* describes the way cells cease to move (and often to divide) as they approach each other and make contact. Cells also exhibit *specific adhesiveness* which permits their aggregation into tissues and the formation of adhering junctions between them. Some cells have isolated cilia which produce directional movement.

Consider the development of nerve and muscle in this context. Chorda-mesoderm induces the formation of a *neural plate* which sinks below the surface and forms a *neural groove*. The lips of the groove fuse, giving a hollow *neural tube* with ciliated cellular walls. Some of these cells divide mitotically (proliferate) and migrate outwards so that the thickness of the wall increases. Simultaneously they differentiate into primitive nerve cells—*neuroblasts*. The presence of a neighbouring mass of mesoderm, the developing *somite*, induces an outgrowth of *nerve fibres* from the neuroblasts. The nerve fibres are guided to and make contact with somite cells, which themselves have gone through phases of proliferation, migration and differentiation into *muscle cells*. Subsequent development of the neural tube and somite are interdependent, the cells of each passing through phases of maturation, growth and functional differentiation.

Mention has been made of the rat/mouse composite (*chimaera*). The use of another chimaera (quail/chick) has been useful in the investigation of other events in morphogenesis and differentiation. In particular it has been possible to follow the migration of *neural crest cells* from alongside the neuraxis to a variety of sites and their differentiation into a variety of cell types. Previously unsuspected derivatives of neural crest have been identified.

Note on the word primitive

As used on this and subsequent pages the word *primitive* means 'first-formed'. It is not always synonymous with *early* which may be taken to imply that subsequent changes are mainly those of time. The changes between *primitive* and *definitive* involve other dimensions and may include changes in constituent parts. *Primitive* is not used here in a phylogenetic sense and has no direct implications about the relationships between so-called higher and lower animals.

Gastrulation

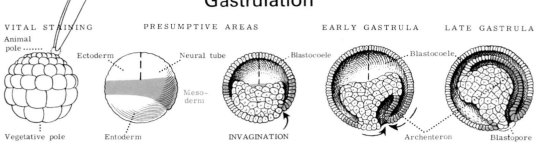

VITAL STAINING

Animal pole ....

Vegetative pole

PRESUMPTIVE AREAS

Ectoderm

Neural tube

Meso-derm

Entoderm

EARLY GASTRULA

Blastocoele

INVAGINATION

Blastocoele

LATE GASTRULA

Blastocoele

Archenteron

Blastopore

Determination

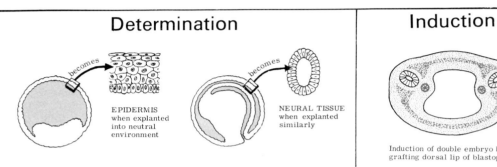

becomes

EPIDERMIS
when explanted
into neutral
environment

becomes

NEURAL TISSUE
when explanted
similarly

Induction

Induction of double embryo by
grafting dorsal lip of blastopore

L S of presumptive neural tube

Cephalic

Caudal

Neural-izing

N   M

CHORDA — MESODERM

Mesoderm-alizing

T S

Neural groove

Somite

Notochord

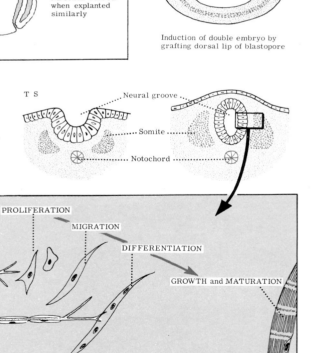

PROLIFERATION

MIGRATION

DIFFERENTIATION

PROLIFERATION

MIGRATION

DIFFERENTIATION

GROWTH and MATURATION

GROWTH and MATURATION

Anomalies

For normal development the genome must be appropriately expressed in time and space so that developmental mechanisms follow their normal course. The genetic aspects of gametogenesis and fertilization, the blocking and deblocking, and the repression and derepression of appropriate parts of the genome and changes in the microenvironment must all occur normally and the gene-controlled synthetic processes must proceed according to a programme.

In this sense cell proliferation, cell death, cell migration and differentiation are all programmed activities. Variations in the programme (the controls) or in the activities (the mechanisms) will result in variety in the developing individual (phenotypic variation). Minor variations are expressed as individual differences but more significant variations are seen as developmental anomalies. The inheritance of differences and anomalies has been considered. The development of these differences or anomalies (*terata*), whether due to genetic or to environmental factors (*teratogens*), depends upon variations in developmental mechanisms. Both genetic and teratogenic effects (*phenocopies*) can be produced whenever developmental mechanisms are operating, i.e. in gametogenesis and in prenatal and postnatal life. However, since development is sequential the earliest aberrations, if uncorrected, will produce the grossest effects (p. 168).

Teratogens

Whilst the number of experimental teratogens are legion, the number of established teratogens in man are limited. Infection of the fetus by the teratogenic *viruses* (rubella and the cytomegaloviruses) may cause abortion, stillbirth, congenital anomaly, disease in infancy or 'late-onset' disease. This they do by disturbing chromosomes, cell division, cell death, fetal vasculature including the placenta and the immune system. Malformations due to rubella (which occur in about 50 per cent of fetuses when infection occurs in the first 2 or 3 weeks of pregnancy and lesser percentages later) may be prevented by the vaccination of susceptible girls. *Ionizing radiation* interferes with cell division and produces cell death but differentiating cells may be particularly sensitive. The gonads should thus not be exposed to non-essential X-rays and, since early pregnancy can only be excluded prior to ovulation, elective diagnostic radiology of the lower abdomen in women should be conducted in the early days of the menstrual cycle. A single 100 mg tablet of the sedative drug *thalidomide* taken by a woman 1 month after conception may result in defec-

tive limb formation in the fetus; the primary cause appears to be damage to the vascular system of the developing limb. The administration of the anticoagulant *warfarin* to a woman may produce fetal anomalies; whether due to local haemorrhage or not is unknown. While deficiency of folic acid, a vitamin of the B group, may be teratogenic *folate antagonists* certainly are: folate deficiency may be responsible for anomalies in children born to *alcoholic* mothers and to *epileptic* mothers on *anticonvulsant* therapy; the folate antagonist aminopterin has been used to produce abortion in the first trimester; if, however, the fetus survived it was grossly deformed. *Steroid hormones* administered to a woman may masculinize her female fetus. *Maternal diseases*, particularly metabolic diseases such as diabetes, may be teratogenic.

Finally there appears to be some unidentified feature of the operating theatre environment which produces an increased incidence of abortion and of congenital anomalies in the families of persons working there.

Whereas these teratogens are known to produce malformations, the status of lysergic acid diethylamide (LSD) is uncertain and many drugs are known to produce less gross aberrations. Thus, for example, *anti-thyroid drugs* may produce congenital goitre, *quinine* may produce deafness, *tetracyclines* stain bones and teeth yellow, and chronic *cigarette smoking* may affect fetal growth. Since the pregnant woman is exposed to so many possibly noxious environmental factors, pronouncements on the teratogenicity of more commonly used drugs are extraordinarily difficult. *The intake of non-essential drugs by pregnant women should be discouraged.*

Superficially, it appears that experimental phenocopies of all known terata can be produced by a variety of teratogens. This suggests that they, and the response of the reacting tissues, are non-specific. However, closer examination reveals that some phenocopies are not identical but differ in detail. For example, a survey of limb malformations before and after the thalidomide era revealed differences: most of the thalidomide babies had an additional malformation of the eye or a midline facial *capillary naevus* (birthmark). There are two further points illustrated by thalidomide. The first is that there is interaction between teratogens and genetic susceptibility: fewer than 25 per cent of the babies of women who took thalidomide at the critical stage of pregnancy were deformed; the remainder showed no detectable sign of ill-effect. The second is that there are wide species differences in teratogenicity: thalidomide produces no detectable effects on fetuses when administered to pregnant rats; other drugs which are teratogenic in rats have not been implicated in the production of human congenital anomalies. Experimental teratogenesis is thus not that helpful in the identification of human teratogens; demonstrated effects in man are the only real criteria. Nevertheless, experimental teratogenesis continues to provide useful information on developmental mechanisms.

Mechanisms

Whatever the aetiological factors, developmental anomalies result from aberrations in developmental mechanisms. At the *cellular level* disturbance of proliferation by interference with cell division or nucleic acid activity may result in paucity or over-production of cells. Disturbance of migration by interference with flow planes, matrix characteristics or ciliary action may result in misdirection or inhibition with consequent defects in morphogenesis. Obviously aberrant differentiation may also produce defects in morphogenesis. Abnormal cell death may result in excessive destruction of cells or in defects of the cavity formation which is necessary for morphogenetic movements.

Similar aberrations also produce predictable effects at the succeeding *tissue level*: these include deficiency or overgrowth of particular tissues. The cell death which is characteristic of, for example, normal joint formation may become excessive and lead to limb shortening whereas failure of cell death may, for example, lead to fused digits. Anomalous contact guidance and/or inhibition and anomalous specific adhesiveness may result in abnormal associations. At the tissue level, moreover, metabolic demands cannot for long be met by simple diffusion, and an effective vascular system becomes necessary. Tissues which suffer oxygen deprivation show local lesions in the form either of fluid-filled blebs or of haemorrhages; these are seen in animals with abnormal genomes as well as those treated with teratogens. Bleb or haematoma formation is followed by unprogrammed cell and tissue death—*necrosis*—which in its turn is followed by *repair* and then by 'catch-up' *redifferentiation*, if the appropriate cell type is available. If it is not available, scar formation, adhesions and secondary effects due to the overgrowth of other tissues may follow. Mechanical factors, such as compression and distraction, may also disturb the organization of tissue. Even at the *organ level*, disturbance of cellular developmental mechanisms can occur as they continue to operate in later fetal and in some cases in postnatal life. In the central nervous system, in particular, differentiation and migration continue into early postnatal life.

Ciliary action appears to be responsible for dextrorotation of the viscera, so that in its absence, asymmetry is random and 50 per cent have *situs inversus*. Also at the *gross level*, in later fetal life there arise alterations in the form of previously normally formed parts—the so-called *congenital postural deformities* (p. 168).

General Vertebrate Development

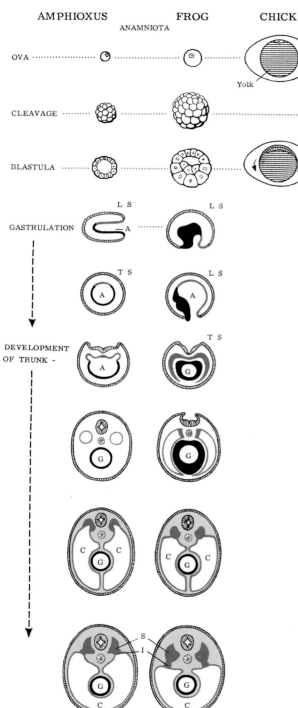

AMPHIOXUS   FROG   CHICK   EUTHERIAN MAMMAL

ANAMNIOTA

OVA

Yolk

CLEAVAGE

BLASTULA

GASTRULATION   L S   L S

DEVELOPMENT OF TRUNK -

KEY

L S	Longitudinal section		
T S	Transverse section		
		G –	Gut
	Ectoderm		
	Mesoderm	I –	Intermediate mesoderm
	Endoderm	S –	Somite
	A – Archenteron		Neural tube
	C – Coelom		Notochord

A lower vertebrate leading an aquatic existence produces many small, yolk-poor—*miolecithal*—eggs which form free-swimming larvae. Most amphibians have larger, more heavily yolked—*mediolecithal*—eggs, which also form free-swimming larvae. In adaption to a terrestrial existence, reptiles and birds produce few, large, yolk-rich—*megalecithal*—eggs, with protective membranes and a shell, and have no larval stage. In eutherian mammals yolk has been secondarily reduced to the miolecithal form, and development occurs in a uterus.

Cleavage of the miolecithal egg of *Amphioxus* forms a simple hollow spherical blastula. The mediolecithal egg of the frog forms a blastula with an eccentric blastocoele surrounded by small animal pole and large vegetative pole blastomeres. During cleavage of the megalecithal egg of the chick, the yolk does not divide. Cytoplasmic divisions are limited to the animal pole, and a bilaminar disc-shaped mass of blastomeres, surmounting the yolk, is produced. A cleft between the laminae may be homologous with the blastocoele of lower forms. A subgerminal cavity filled with nutritive liquefying yolk soon forms between the blastomeres and the main yolk mass. Cleavage of the miolecithal egg of a eutherian mammal forms a solid *morula* which soon cavitates and becomes a hollow blastocyst with an eccentrically placed *inner cell mass.* Cleavage is said to be *complete* or *incomplete* according to the extent of cytoplasmic subdivision, and to be *equal* or *unequal* according to the relative size of the early blastomeres. More important in subsequent development, however, are the different nucleocytoplasmic relationships in the blastomeres produced by division of a zygote with regional differences in its cytoplasm.

In forms with free-swimming larvae (*Anamniota*) the whole of the blastula is transformed into the embryo, whereas in terrestrial forms (*Amniota*) some of the blastula forms extraembryonic membranes.

In *Amphioxus*, gastrulation proceeds by invagination of the presumptive endoderm and chorda-mesoderm with obliteration of the blastocoele. The resulting archenteron has a roof of chorda-mesoderm in contact with presumptive neural tube, but is lined elsewhere with endoderm in contact with ectoderm. Further development of the trunk involves induction of a neural plate which rolls up and sinks below the surface ectoderm, forming the neural tube. The chorda-mesoderm separates from the endoderm and forms an axial notochord underlying the neural tube, and, more laterally, a series of paired *coelomic pouches*. The circumferential continuity of the endoderm is restored with the formation of a tube—the definitive gut. The paired coelomic pouches, which flank the notochord, form the basis of the *metameric* segmentation which characterizes chordates. They expand dorsally and ventrally to form *bilateral coelomic cavities* (CC) separated by the gut and its dorsal and ventral mesenteries. The ventral mesentery and intersegmental partitions subsequently break down, forming a *single coelomic cavity* (C). The walls of the coelomic pouches thus give rise to a layer of *splanchnic* mesoderm surrounding gut endoderm, and a layer of *somatic* mesoderm lining the ectoderm. Much of the somatic mesoderm forms segmental body-wall musculature and is in part homologous with the

mesodermal somite of higher forms.

In the frog (mediolecithal egg) gastrulation differs somewhat, but formation of the neural tube, notochord and gut is generally similar to that of *Amphioxus*. However, during notochord formation, the mesoderm temporarily forms a solid layer, intervening between endoderm and ectoderm. This extends ventrally and, later, cavitates so that splanchnic and somatic layers of mesoderm enclose bilateral coelomic cavities. The ventral mesentery later disappears with confluence of the coelomic cavities. Alongside the notochord the mesoderm forms metamerically arranged somites. More laterally is a strip of *intermediate mesoderm*, which will give rise to the kidneys and gonads.

The foregoing accounts of trunk development can be applied, with some modification, to the whole of the phylum *Chordata*. The principal modifications are associated with varying amounts of yolk and the presence of extraembryonic membranes. At comparable stages in their development all vertebrates have certain features in common, and these may be recognized at appropriate stages in human development.

Generalized Vertebrate

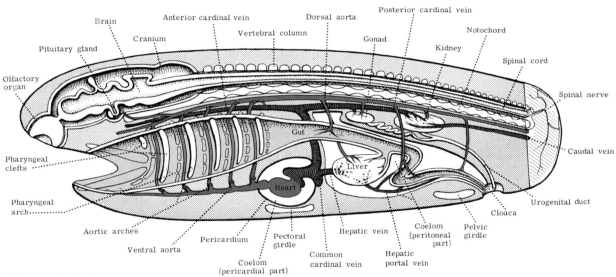

Note particularly:

1 The hollow dorsal nervous system expanded cranially to form a brain.
2 The brain-case and segmented vertebral column.
3 The relationship of the notochord to brain-case, vertebral column, pituitary gland, dorsal aorta and gut.
4 The pharynx with its arches separated by clefts or grooves, each arch containing a skeletal support, muscles, nerves and an aortic arch connecting dorsal and ventral aortae.

5 The mouth in series with these pharyngeal clefts, the jaws being the skeletal supports of the first arch.
6 The ventral tubular heart in the pericardial part of the coelomic cavity which is receiving blood from the common cardinal vein and liver caudally and passing it via a ventral aorta to aortic arches.
7 The gut and urogenital duct opening into a common cloaca.

29

Extraembryonic membranes

Trunk formation is essentially similar in the *Anamniota* (e.g. *Amphioxus* and frog) and *Amniota* (reptiles, birds and mammals). The latter, however, derive their name from the possession of extraembryonic membranes. The eggs of reptiles and birds are adapted for laying on dry land. They are heavily yolked and possess a hard shell. The membranes they develop provide a local aquatic environment for the embryo and facilities for respiratory exchange, segregation of waste products and assimilation of the yolk. In mammals the membranes are modified and development occurs in a uterus.

The chick blastula is a bilaminar disc of blastomeres surmounting the yolk. The margins of this disc proliferate and spread until the yolk is almost completely enclosed. Meanwhile trunk formation proceeds and mesoderm produced within the body of the embryo spreads to give a trilaminar membrane around the yolk. The three laminae are endoderm, mesoderm and ectoderm. Cavities appear in the extraembryonic mesoderm and coalesce to form an *extraembryonic coelom* which is continuous at the lateral edge of the embryonic disc with an *intraembryonic coelom*. The walls of the coelom are the *somatopleure* (ectoderm + somatic mesoderm) and the *splanchnopleure* (endoderm + splanchnic mesoderm).

Somatopleure

The intraembryonic somatopleure forms the body wall and limbs. As the yolk mass is reduced the embryo sinks, and folds of the extraembryonic somatopleure surround the embryo. The folds meet dorsal to the embryo, thus enclosing a cavity and subdividing the extraembryonic somatopleure into two membranes: the *amnion* surrounds the amniotic cavity, which becomes filled with amniotic fluid; the *chorion* lines the shell and shell membrane.

Splanchnopleure

The intraembryonic splanchnopleure forms the *gut* and its derivatives. The extraembryonic splanchnopleure covers the yolk mass as the *yolk sac* and develops a diverticulum—the *allantois*—which grows into the extraembryonic coelom. The allantois expands, almost filling the extraembryonic coelom, and its outer wall eventually fuses with the chorion, forming an allantochorionic membrane.

The amniotic fluid eliminates gravitational stresses, the formation of adhesions and the danger of desiccation. Blood vessels in the wall of the yolk sac transport nutrients derived from the yolk, to the embryo. Blood vessels in the wall of the expanding allantois vascularize the overlying chorion. Respiratory exchanges occur between the vascularized membranes and the external air via the porous shell. The cavity of the allantois serves as a receptacle for fetal urine.

Although the mammalian egg is miolecithal, and development proceeds in a uterus, extraembryonic membranes are formed which resemble those formed from a megalecithal egg. This suggests that mammals have evolved from species possessing megalecithal eggs. However, mammalian yolk reserves are poor, and some part of the extraembryonic membranes comes into close apposition with uterine tissues so that physiological exchanges between mother and embryo can occur, i.e. a *placenta* is formed. Exchanges occur between the embryonic and the maternal bloodstreams, which are separated by a placental membrane of varying constitution.

The developing sheep embryo has an amnion (formed by folding), a chorion (in apposition with uterine tissues) and a splanchnopleuric yolk sac (containing no yolk and in part incorporated into the body as the gut). From the caudal part of the gut a splanchnopleuric diverticulum—the allantois—grows and expands in the extraembryonic coelom. The allantois and its blood vessels fuse with the chorion and establish the embryonic part of a *chorioallantoic placenta*.

In man, the definitive amnion is formed by folding after cavitation of the inner cell mass. An extensive extraembryonic coelom is formed early and contains a small splanchnopleuric yolk sac. The endodermal allantois is small, but allantoic mesoderm extends to the inner aspect of the chorion as the *connecting stalk*. Allantoic blood vessels, formed in the *connecting stalk*, vascularize the chorionic part of the human placenta (which is thus also classified as chorioallantoic).

In other mammals the embryonic aspect of the placenta may be vascularized by yolk sac (*vitelline*) vessels. A simple yolk sac placenta occurs typically in marsupials, and transiently in many Eutheria. Rodents generally exhibit some form of inverted yolk sac placenta. In the incomplete form, the vascularized embryonic half of the yolk sac is apposed to the non-vascular abembryonic half which, in its turn, is apposed to maternal tissues. In the complete form, disappearance of the abembryonic half exposes the endoderm of the vascularized embryonic half and allows contact between it and maternal tissues.

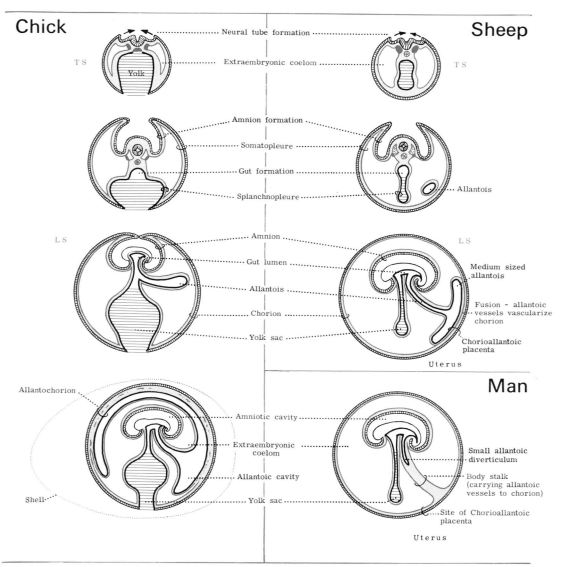

Chick

Sheep

- Neural tube formation
- Extraembryonic coelom
- Yolk
- T S
- Amnion formation
- Somatopleure
- Gut formation
- Splanchnopleure
- Allantois
- L S
- Amnion
- Gut lumen
- Allantois
- Chorion
- Yolk sac
- Medium sized allantois
- Fusion - allantoic vessels vascularize chorion
- Chorioallantoic placenta
- Uterus

Man

- Allantochorion
- Amniotic cavity
- Extraembryonic coelom
- Allantoic cavity
- Yolk sac
- Shell
- Small allantoic diverticulum
- Body stalk (carrying allantoic vessels to chorion)
- Site of Chorioallantoic placenta
- Uterus

Mammalian Placentation

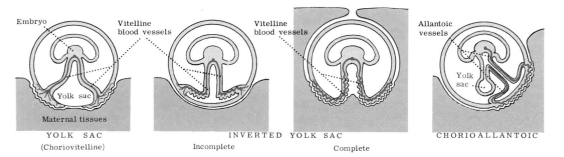

Embryo	Vitelline blood vessels	Vitelline blood vessels	Allantoic vessels
Yolk sac			Yolk sac
Maternal tissues			
YOLK SAC (Choriovitelline)	INVERTED YOLK SAC		CHORIOALLANTOIC
	Incomplete	Complete	

Gametogenesis, Fertilization and Implantation

Gametogenesis is the formation of the germ cells or *gametes* and entails *meiosis* or *reduction division*. Each gamete thus contains only 23 chromosomes—i.e. only half the hereditary information necessary for the development of a new individual.

The male gametes or *spermatozoa* are formed in the *testes* which are located in the scrotum. From each testis, spermatozoa pass via a *ductus (vas) deferens* to the groin and thence to the *prostate* gland at the base of the bladder. The *urethra*, which leads from the bladder through the prostate and along the penis, is a common passage for urine from the bladder and semen from each side. *Semen* contains spermatozoa and secretions from various glands along the path from the testis, including the prostate.

The female gametes or *ova* are formed in the *ovaries* which are located in the pelvis. During the reproductive period of a woman's life her ovaries produce ova in cycles, each lasting about 28 days. In the first half of each *ovarian cycle*, germ cells ripen and come to occupy fluid-filled sacs or *follicles* in the ovary. One of these follicles, outstripping the others, matures and ruptures thus releasing its ovum (*ovulation*) on about the 14th day of the cycle. The other follicles then shrivel up (*atrophy*). The ruptured follicle forms a yellow body—the *corpus luteum*. This grows for some days but then, in the absence of pregnancy, atrophies and a new cycle begins. In the first (*follicular*) half of the cycle the ovary secretes female sex hormones called *oestrogens*; in the second (*luteal*) half its corpus luteum secretes oestrogens and a second female sex hormone—*progesterone*. The secretion of these hormones in the ovarian cycle produces a cycle of changes in the lining of the uterus (the *endometrium*) which is called the *menstrual cycle*.

The first half of the menstrual cycle begins with the endometrium being shed at *menstruation*. Under the influence of oestrogens, it is then rebuilt and thickens. After ovulation, under the influence of oestrogens and progesterone, the endometrium becomes yet thicker, becomes spongy and accumulates nutrients so that it is ready to receive a fertilized ovum. It is said to be *progestational*. If a fertilized ovum does not arrive, the corpus luteum atrophies and the influences of oestrogens and progesterone are withdrawn. As a result, the endometrium is shed in the *menses* at the beginning of the next cycle.

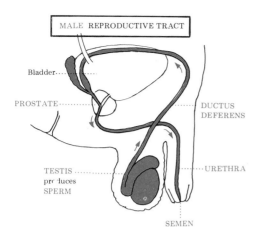

MALE REPRODUCTIVE TRACT

Bladder

PROSTATE

DUCTUS DEFERENS

TESTIS produces SPERM

URETHRA

SEMEN

FEMALE REPRODUCTIVE TRACT (non-pregnant)

UTERINE TUBE

OVUM

UTERUS

Developing FOLLICLE

ENDOMETRIUM shed monthly in the MENSES

OVARY

FERTILIZATION CLEAVAGE IMPLANTATION

Path of CONCEPTUS after fertilization

IMPLANTATION in thickening ENDOMETRIUM

FERTILIZATION of ovum by SPERM

Path of SPERM before fertilization

For fertilization to occur a *spermatozoon* must swim up the cavity of the uterus and along the *uterine tube* to meet and penetrate an *ovum* which has been shed at ovulation. The resulting single fertilized cell or *zygote* has 46 chromosomes (i.e. the full amount of hereditary information necessary for the development of a new individual). The zygote divides into two cells. This and subsequent divisions are by *mitosis* so that the number of chromosomes is maintained and hereditary information is passed on unchanged. Division of cells continues during passage of the *conceptus* down the uterine tube. As a result the mass of cells which reaches the uterus looks like a miniature mulberry. The layer of cells on its outside will be concerned with nutrition of the conceptus and forms the *trophoblast* (Gk *trophe* = nutrition). The embryo will form from cells inside that outer layer. They become pushed to one side by a fluid-filled cavity and are then referred to as the *inner cell mass*. The trophoblast and the enclosed cavity and inner cell mass constitute the *blastocyst*.

About a week after fertilization the trophoblast over the inner cell mass erodes the endometrium so that the blastocyst comes to lie in an *implantation cavity*, most commonly on the posterior wall of the uterus. The trophoblast also secretes a hormone which acts on the ovary and causes the corpus luteum to persist in the first half of pregnancy. As a result it continues to secrete oestrogens and progesterone; under their influence the endometrium accumulates more nutrients for the support of the conceptus and because it is shed with the afterbirth is then known as the *decidua*.

GAMETOGENESIS

From the GONADS

TESTES   or   OVARIES

cells containing 46 chromosomes divide by MEIOSIS (or reduction division) to form the GAMETES each with 23 chromosomes

SPERMS   or   OVA

on fertilization the new individual

a ZYGOTE

has 46 chromosomes

About 5 days after conception

TROPHOBLAST

Cavity

Inner cell mass in which the EMBRYO will form

BLASTOCYST

Spermatogenesis

The primary sex organ (*gonad*) in the male is the *testis*. It is enclosed by an isolated part of the coelomic membrane—the *tunica vaginalis*—and has a tough fibrous capsule—the *tunica albuginea*—which sends septa into the organ, dividing it into lobules. Each *lobule* is occupied by one to three coiled *seminiferous tubules* which form a series of closed loops. Each loop drains, via a *straight tubule*, into a network of channels—the *rete testis*—which occupies a posterior thickening of the tunica albuginea. Between the seminiferous tubules are plexuses of capillaries and lymphatics, autonomic nerve fibres and groups of rounded *interstitial (Leydig) cells* which produce the steroid sex hormone—testosterone.

The epithelium of the seminiferous tubule has a basement membrane on which lie germinal cells called spermatogonia, and *Sertoli (sustentacular) cells*; the Sertoli cells produce a substance—*androgen-binding protein* (ABP)—which binds testosterone to structures concerned with sperm formation and maturation. Between neighbouring Sertoli cells there are tight and gap junctional complexes which constitute a blood–testis barrier and separate a *basal compartment* containing spermatogonia from an *adluminal compartment* containing their derivatives. The activity of the seminiferous epithelium is cyclical, each cycle lasting 16 days and resulting in daughter cells which remain connected by cytoplasmic bridges. In the basal compartment the population of spermatogonia is maintained by proliferative mitoses. After quantal mitoses some spermatogonia enter the first of the four cycles taken for maturation to spermatozoa: their daughter cells pass from the basal into the adluminal compartment where they are seen as large joined spherical *primary spermatocytes* embedded in the sides of adjacent Sertoli cells. The second and third cycles are spent on the divisions of meiosis, each primary spermatocyte producing two *secondary spermatocytes* and thence four smaller (still joined) *spermatids*. In the process the chromosomal content is reduced from the diploid to the haploid number, genetic material is redistributed, and the X and Y chromosomes are segregated. The fourth cycle is spent on the metamorphosis from spermatid to *spermatozoon*: the spermatid has now reached the luminal end of the Sertoli cell; the nucleus of the spermatid condenses and forms most of the sperm head; an *acrosomal cap* is derived from the Golgi apparatus; the centrioles move to the back of the head; an *axoneme* grows back from the distal centriole and projects beyond the general cell surface; mitochondria align and form a helical sheath around the proximal part of the axoneme; finally most of the cytoplasm is shed.

A mature sperm presents a head, neck and tail. The ovoid *head* is flattened anteriorly and appears pear-shaped in profile. It is bounded by a cell membrane continuous with that of the neck and tail. Underlying it, over the anterior two-thirds of the head, is the acrosomal cap, and over the posterior one-third, the nuclear membrane. The chromosomes retain their identity within the sperm head. In the *neck*, the *connecting piece*—a series of nine segmented columns joined to each other and the nucleus—surrounds the remaining proximal centriole, the distal one having disappeared. The axoneme to which the distal centriole gave rise consists of a central pair of microtubules surrounded by a ring of nine doublet microtubules. For the greater part of its length the axoneme is surrounded by nine outer dense fibres which are joined to the nine segmented columns of the connecting piece. The *tail* consists of a middle piece, a principal part and an end piece: surrounding the longitudinal elements in the *middle piece* is the helical mitochondrial sheath which ends at a ring; surrounding the *principal part* is a fibrous sheath incorporating two of the nine outer dense fibres and surrounding the others; the *end piece* consists only of axoneme surrounded by cell membrane. The sperm head contains the genetic apparatus and its coverings produce secretions which facilitate fertilization. The remainder of the sperm is locomotor in function, the mitochondrial sheath being concerned with energy production and the axoneme and its surrounding fibres being a complex system of contractile proteins.

Spermatogenesis does not proceed simultaneously in all parts of the testis or even in all parts of the same tubule; shorter or longer stretches of resting tubule alternate with short patches of active epithelium. From the tubules the sperm-containing fluid is passed through the straight tubules, which are lined by fat-laden Sertoli cells, to the rete testis, where the epithelium is predominantly low columnar. The sperms then enter the *efferent ductules*, which become increasingly coiled as they lead to the *head of the epididymis*. Some of the columnar lining cells are ciliated, others bear microvilli and a single flagellum. The cilia and flagella, assisted by intermittent contraction of the smooth muscle present in the walls, impart movement to the sperm-containing fluid which is concentrated in passage.

The Testis

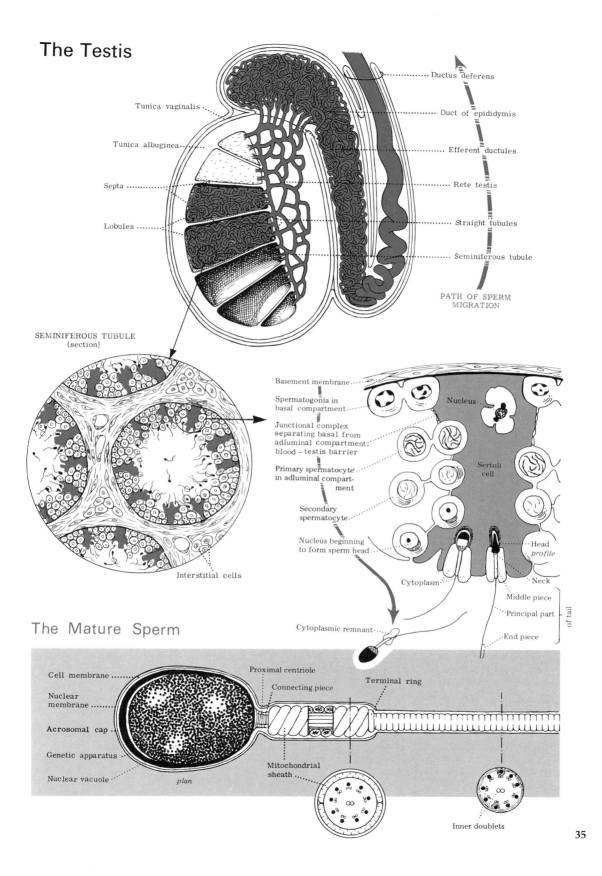

Tunica vaginalis

Tunica albuginea

Septa

Lobules

Ductus deferens

Duct of epididymis

Efferent ductules

Rete testis

Straight tubules

Seminiferous tubule

PATH OF SPERM
MIGRATION

SEMINIFEROUS TUBULE
(section)

Interstitial cells

Basement membrane

Spermatogonia in
basal compartment

Junctional complex
separating basal from
adluminal compartment:
blood – testis barrier

Primary spermatocyte
in adluminal compart-
ment

Secondary
spermatocyte

Nucleus beginning
to form sperm head

Cytoplasm

Nucleus

Sertoli
cell

Head
profile

Neck

Middle piece

Principal part

of tail

End piece

Cytoplasmic remnant

The Mature Sperm

Cell membrane

Nuclear
membrane

Acrosomal cap

Genetic apparatus

Nuclear vacuole

Proximal centriole

Connecting piece

Terminal ring

Mitochondrial
sheath

plan

Inner doublets

Sperm transport

From the efferent ductules the sperm-containing fluid is passed into the long tortuous *duct of the epididymis,* which is lined by a secretory epithelium of columnar cells with non-motile stereocilia. Secretions arise from the cytoplasm between the stereocilia and assist the nutrition and maturation of the sperms during their slow passage through the epididymis. The *tail of the epididymis* forms the principal storehouse for sperms awaiting ejaculation. Thereafter, the convolutions cease and a similar epithelium continues as the lining of the proximal part of the *ductus (vas) deferens.* The stereocilia are absent from the distal part of the ductus, including the terminal *ampulla.* Transport through the epididymis and ductus deferens is due to the peristaltic contraction of the smooth muscle in their walls. The ampullary mucous membrane is highly folded, forming a complex system of spaces which accumulates secretions and functions as a secondary sperm store. The ampulla narrows rapidly and unites with the *excretory duct of the seminal vesicle* to form an *ejaculatory duct.* In the seminal vesicle of each side a series of blind diverticula open into a convoluted tube which ends in a straight excretory duct. The diverticula are lined with a columnar secretory epithelium, which produces a viscous secretion rich in fructose and a wide variety of prostaglandins. The two ejaculatory ducts, which traverse the *prostate,* have a lining of secretory columnar epithelium with glandular evaginations and open into the prostatic *urethra.* The prostatic, membranous and penile urethra as far as the fossa terminalis, are lined with a transitional epithelium and receive secretions from further accessory glands. These include the *prostate,* the *prostatic utricle,* the *bulbourethral glands,* and other small *urethral glands.* The alkaline prostatic secretion is serous and has been shown to contain acid phosphatase, citrates, zinc, magnesium and the unique amines spermine and spermidine.

During coitus the seminal fluid is ejaculated into the vagina. The reflex process of ejaculation may be divided into two phases: in the first—emission—contraction of smooth muscle delivers the various components of semen into the posterior urethra; in the second—ejaculation proper—the striped muscle of the urogenital diaphragm (particularly the bulbocavernosus muscle) contracts spasmodically and expels the seminal fluid from the urethra. The accessory glands do not deliver their secretions to the urethra simultaneously. Initially the urethral and bulbourethral and prostate glands produce a small amount of pre-ejaculatory fluid. Next come the sperm-bearing secretions from the ductus deferens, the epididymis and the testis itself. The last part has the highest content of fructose, which comes only from the seminal vesicles and is the prime source of energy for ejaculated sperms.

During its development and storage a sperm is non-motile and is supported by secretions from the various epithelia and hydrolysis of the membrane of its cytoplasmic remnant. The non-motile condition of the sperm may be due to an accumulation of acid metabolites during storage. This would be diluted at emission by the alkaline secretions of the accessory sex glands. The secretions also tend to neutralize and remove the inhibitory effect of the acid content of the male urethra and the vagina. The fructose contributed by the seminal vesicles is probably broken down by the enzyme systems of the mitochondrial sheath of the sperm with the liberation of the energy necessary for its highly motile state after ejaculation. The fertilizing power and potential motility of sperms recovered from the head of the epididymis are low or absent but they increase progressively during the slow passage of the sperms through the epididymis.

The *ejaculate* (average 3.5 ml, normal range 2–6 ml) consists of spermatozoa suspended in the secretion of the accessory glands and genital passages—the *seminal plasma.* The average density of sperms is 100 million/ml (normal range 60–150 million/ml) and, of these, 20–25 per cent are abnormal forms (e.g. double or small heads or tails) and over 75 per cent are motile. The sperms are capable of moving 2–3 mm per minute, but the actual speed varies with the pH of their environment. As noted, they are non-motile during storage, but become highly motile in the ejaculate. Their velocity is probably quite slow in the acid vagina (perhaps 0.5 mm per minute) but increases after reaching the alkaline environment of the uterine cavity. Semen is rich in the enzyme hyaluronidase which is an important 'spreading factor', and causes lysis of intercellular substance. It facilitates the approach of the sperm towards the ovum through its covering layers of cells.

Some 20 per cent of marriages are unintentionally childless after 5 years; it is estimated that the cause in one-third to one-half is male infertility. This may be associated with endocrine disorders, defective spermatogenesis or obstruction of the genital ducts. Semen analysis may reveal a low seminal volume (< 2 ml) or a low sperm count (< 20 million/ml). For potential fertility at least 40 per cent of the spermatozoa should be motile after 2 hours and some should remain motile for 24 hours. The percentage of abnormal forms of spermatozoa should be less than 40 per cent.

Enzyme deficiency in the semen and unfavourable conditions in the cervix may be revealed by Huhner's test in which the cervical mucus is examined after coitus.

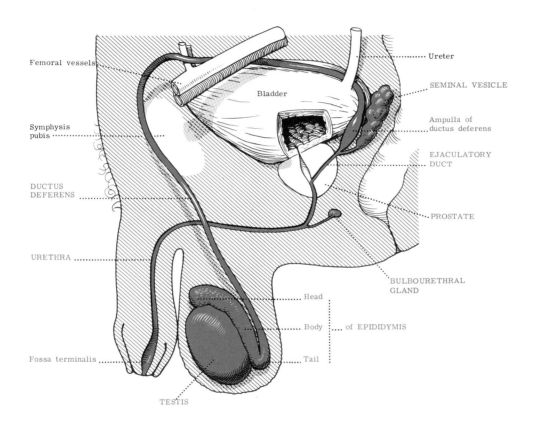

Femoral vessels

Symphysis
pubis

DUCTUS
DEFERENS

URETHRA

Fossa terminalis

TESTIS

Bladder

Ureter

SEMINAL VESICLE

Ampulla of
ductus deferens

EJACULATORY
DUCT

PROSTATE

BULBOURETHRAL
GLAND

Head

Body   of EPIDIDYMIS

Tail

Female genital tract

The *vagina* is essentially a fibromuscular tube lined by a stratified squamous epithelium. It undergoes slight changes in thickness, keratinization and glycogen content under the cyclical influence of ovarian hormones, and is lubricated by cervical mucus which contains leucocytes and desquamated epithelial cells. The normal bacterial flora of the vagina includes a lactobacillus which degrades glycogen to lactic acid, producing the characteristic acid reaction of the vaginal fluid—pH 3.8 to 4.5.

The vaginal epithelium is continued over the *cervix uteri* to the *external os*. The mucosa of the *cervical canal* is ridged and covered with a tall columnar mucus-secreting epithelium which extends into large branched tubular glands. Ovarian hormones have little effect on the structure of the mucosa but the secretion of alkaline mucus (favourable to the sperm) is increased near ovulation time. At the *internal os* is a region transitional between the mucosa lining the cervix and the *endometrium* lining the *body* and *fundus* of the *uterus*.

Soon after menstruation the *endometrium* consists of a cubical mucus-secreting epithelium with simple tubular glands and a cellular stroma bearing arteries and a venous network. Under the influence of ovarian hormones the whole endometrium undergoes dramatic changes which constitute the menstrual cycle. Outside the endometrium, and blending with it, is the smooth muscle coat—the *myometrium*.

The mucous membrane of the *uterine tube* is thrown into a complicated series of folds which subdivide the lumen into fine intercommunicating spaces. The folds are most highly developed at the ampullary end of the tube where they continue as the *fimbriae*. Two types of columnar epithelial cell are present throughout the tube, secretory cells predominating at the uterine end and ciliated cells at the ampullary end. Under the influence of ovarian hormones the cells undergo cyclical changes. They increase in size during the first half of the menstrual cycle and reach a maximum at ovulation time. Thereafter the secretory cells become active and the ciliated cells retrogress.

Oogenesis

The primary sex organ (gonad) in the female is the *ovary*. It has a small vascular *medulla* covered by a thick *cortex*. It is limited externally by a poorly defined *tunica albuginea* covered by a *cuboidal epithelium* which is continuous at the hilum, with the squamous

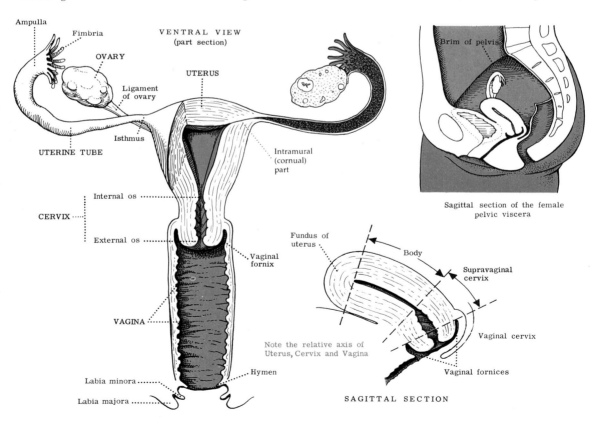

Ampulla
Fimbria
OVARY
VENTRAL VIEW
(part section)
UTERUS
Ligament
of ovary
Isthmus
UTERINE TUBE
Intramural
(cornual)
part
Internal os
CERVIX
External os
Vaginal
fornix
VAGINA
Labia minora
Labia majora
Hymen

Brim of pelvis

Sagittal section of the female
pelvic viscera

Fundus of
uterus
Body
Supravaginal
cervix
Vaginal cervix
Vaginal fornices
Note the relative axis of
Uterus, Cervix and Vagina

SAGITTAL SECTION

epithelium lining the peritoneal cavity elsewhere. Oogenesis proceeds in the cortex, where germinal elements, in varying stages of maturity, are embedded in a vascular fibrocellular *stroma*.

The ovarian cortex contains *primordial follicles* which consist of a large spherical *primary oocyte* (derived from a primordial sex cell) surrounded by a group of flattened *pregranulosa cells*. The primary oocyte accumulates a crescentic mass of mitochondria and fat globules in its cytoplasm, and the nucleus becomes eccentric. Meanwhile the pregranulosa cells divide mitotically and produce a mass of small rounded *granulosa cells*. These secrete a hyaline *zona pellucida* around the oocyte. As the oocyte approaches maximal size, fluid-filled spaces appear between the granulosa cells and coalesce to form a *follicular cavity*. This separates the parietal cells of the *membrana granulosa* from those which surround the oocyte (later termed the *corona radiata*). The follicle increases rapidly in size by cellular division and by accumulation of fluid. As this occurs the surrounding stromal cells differentiate into a fibrocellular *theca externa* and a vascular *theca interna*. The ripening follicle approaches the surface of the ovary and increasing distension leads to rupture. The oocyte, its zona pellucida and corona radiata become detached from the follicular wall and escape from the ovary—*ovulation.*

All the oocytes which the ovaries will ever have, approximately 2 million, are present in early meiosis at birth. Vast numbers undergo atresia in infancy and childhood; only about 300 000 are present at the age of 7 years. Fewer than 400 reach maturity and are ovulated.

As the follicle develops, the primary oocyte completes the first meiotic division with the extrusion of a small nuclear mass—the *first polar body* or *polocyte.* During this division the chromosomes are reduced from the diploid to the haploid number and most of the cytoplasm is retained by the *secondary oocyte.* A second maturation spindle is soon formed and ovulation occurs. Completion of the second meiotic division, with final redistribution of genetic material and the production of a *second polar body*, is initiated by sperm penetration.

After ovulation the collapsed follicle is transformed into an endocrine gland—the *corpus luteum.* The theca externa forms a connective tissue capsule and trabeculae which bear theca interna derivatives (blood vessels and small *thecoluteal cells*) into the substance of the gland. Between the trabeculae the granulosa cells are modified to form large, polyhedral, vacuolated *granulosoluteal* cells containing the carotenoid pigment *lutein.*

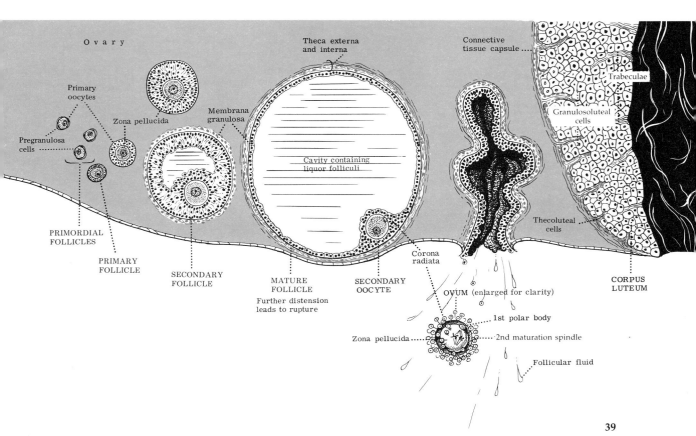

39

Female reproductive cycles

All parts of the female genital tract exhibit periodic changes in structure and function. The changes affecting the vagina, uterine cervix and uterine tubes are relatively slight. The more profound changes of the non-pregnant endometrium constitute the *menstrual cycle* and those of the ovary, the *ovarian cycle*. The latter includes the phasic production of ovarian sex hormones which cause the changes throughout the rest of the genital tract. The ovarian cycle is under the rhythmic endocrine control of the *adenohypophysis* and this, in its turn, is dominated by the influence of the *central nervous system*.

Pituitary gonadotrophins

A decapeptide *gonadotrophin-releasing hormone* (GnRH) is produced by the hypothalamus and reaches the adenohypophysis via the hypophyseal portal system. Under the influence of GnRH the adenohypophysis releases gonad-stimulating hormones. *Follicle-stimulating hormone* (FSH) and *luteinizing hormone* (LH) are glycoproteins, evidently both stored in granules in the basophil cells of the adenohypophysis.

In the female, FSH stimulates the development of ovarian follicles and thus promotes oogenesis. However, follicles can develop up to the beginning of cavity formation without pituitary stimulation. FSH induces little, if any, hormone production, but its release from the adenohypophysis is inhibited by a group of steroid hormones—the *oestrogens*. In the male, FSH stimulates synthesis of androgen-binding protein (ABP) by Sertoli cells and thus promotes spermatogenesis.

In the female, LH has five actions, all dependent upon prior action of FSH:

1 It furthers the ripening of follicles.
2 It stimulates rupture of the ripe follicle—*ovulation*.
3 It stimulates the differentiation of granulosa cells and theca interna cells to granulosoluteal and thecoluteal cells respectively—*luteinization*—thus inducing corpus luteum formation.
4 It stimulates the granulosoluteal cells to produce *progesterone*—also a steroid hormone.
5 It stimulates the theca interna cells, and their derivatives the thecoluteal cells, to produce *oestrogens*.

The release of LH from the adenohypophysis is promoted by physiological increases in oestrogens, and is inhibited by progesterone. Certainly, large doses of progesterone and oestrogen in combination, as in oral contraceptives, block the release of gonadotrophins and thus prevent ovulation. In the male, LH stimulates the interstitial cells of the testis to produce the androgen *testosterone*.

Prolactin (PRL), which is a straight-chain polypeptide and not a glycoprotein, is important in luteinization in the rat but not in man. In the human female it stimulates the mammary glands, which have previously been prepared by oestrogens and progesterone, to produce milk. A hypothalamic *prolactin-inhibiting factor* (PIF) and high doses of oestrogens inhibit the release of PRL from the adenohypophysis: suckling suppresses PIF, thus stimulating PRL secretion and lactation; high doses of oestrogens are used to suppress lactation. The action of PRL in the male is unknown.

The ovarian cycle

The recurring processes of *oogenesis, corpus luteum formation* and *ovarian hormone production* constitute the ovarian cycle. Except during pregnancy, ovarian cycles persist throughout the normal reproductive life of the female. It is convenient to divide each cycle into two phases—an initial *follicular phase* and a postovulatory *luteal phase*. Usually an ovarian cycle lasts 26–30 days, its luteal phase lasting some 13–15 days. Cycles of longer or shorter duration are due to variation in the length of the follicular phase.

During the *follicular phase* a number of young ovarian follicles begin to grow, probably being self-regulated by their own oestrogens acting locally. Some of these follicles develop cavities and continue to enlarge under the influence of FSH. Normally, however, only one follicle ripens fully and ruptures. For ovulation to occur the balanced activity of both FSH and LH is necessary. The less ripe follicles undergo atresia—the follicle collapses, the oocyte and granulosa cells degenerate and the cavity is obliterated by fibrous tissue. The surrounding theca interna cells differentiate into the small, rounded, *interstitial cells* of the ovary. The oestrogens, which are steroid hormones, are mainly produced by theca interna cells, although the interstitial cells and the stroma generally may be concerned. Early in the follicular phase the secretion of small amounts of oestrogen promotes the release of LH from the adenohypophysis. This, in its turn, increases the secretion of oestrogens which stimulates GnRH production and reduces its pituitary threshold so that the levels of LH and oestrogen steadily build up. The increasing level of oestrogens also inhibits the release of FSH so that, after the oestrogens have reached their peak, LH shows a greater relative rise than FSH, and stimulates ovulation. There is usually a drop, followed by a sustained rise, in body temperature at ovulation time.

The Female Reproductive Cycles

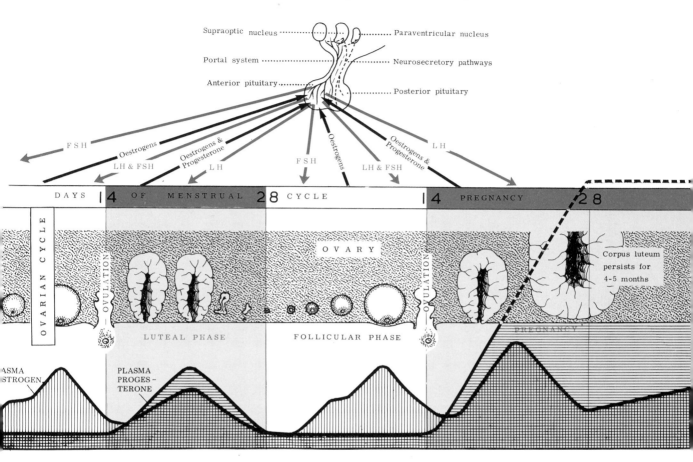

The *luteal phase* follows ovulation and a corpus luteum is formed as LH stimulates the luteinization of the granulosa and theca interna cells to granulosoluteal and thecoluteal cells respectively. The thecoluteal cells probably continue to secrete oestrogens while the granulosoluteal cells produce progesterone. The rising levels of oestrogen and progesterone now inhibit GnRH production and the release of further pituitary gonadotrophic hormones, which not only prevents further ovulation in the same cycle but also leads to a fall in the levels of oestrogen and progesterone and the initiation of a new cycle. If the ovum is not fertilized, it is lost at menstruation: the corpus luteum of menstruation reaches maturity and is secreting maximally by the 21st day; it then probably autonomously begins to retrogress. It is ultimately replaced by a small fibrous cicatrix—the corpus albi-

cans. If fertilization occurs, the corpus luteum of pregnancy increases in size and remains functionally active throughout the first 4–5 months of pregnancy.

Human chorionic gonadotrophin

A glycoprotein similar in structure and function to LH, *human chorionic gonadotrophin* (hCG) is secreted by the *trophoblast*. Its release may be controlled by a locally produced GnRH. First appearing early in pregnancy, hCG attains a peak level in the first trimester, and then falls off. The role of hCG is to keep the corpus luteum secreting until the developing placenta can assume the production of the oestrogens and progesterone necessary to pregnancy.

The menstrual cycle

Changes in oestrogen and progesterone levels produce the endometrial changes of the menstrual cycle, which thus also lasts 26–30 days. The days of the cycle are numbered from the first day of the menstrual flow, which lasts 3–5 days. In a cycle of 28 days, ovulation occurs on or about the 14th day. In cycles of longer or shorter duration, because of the relative constancy of the luteal phase, ovulation usually occurs 13–15 days before the onset of the succeeding menstrual period.

The oestrogens of the follicular phase produce a *proliferative phase* in the endometrium and an increase in the contractile proteins and contractions of the myometrium. After ovulation the oestrogens and progesterone of the luteal phase produce a *secretory phase* in the endometrium and inhibit the contractions of the myometrium. These are the changes which prepare the uterus for the reception and maintenance of a fertilized ovum.

Soon after menstruation the endometrium is thin and has a cubical epithelium. This dips into simple tubular glands which reach the myometrium. Between the glands a dense stroma of spindle-shaped cells is pervaded by blood vessels. During the *proliferative (oestrogenic) phase* the endometrium thickens and shows an increase in water content, vascularity, protein content and enzyme activity. The epithelium becomes columnar. The superficial and deep parts of the glands remain straight, but the intermediate parts become slightly tortuous and produce a little serous secretion. The stroma exhibits three strata—a dense stratum compactum between the straight necks of the glands, a dense stratum basale between the straight bases of the glands, and an oedematous loosely packed stratum spongiosum between these two layers. The arteries supplying the endometrium are of two types: short straight arteries to the stratum basale, and longer spiral arteries to the more superficial strata. Drainage to the uterine veins is via a complex venous network.

During the *secretory (progestational) phase* the endometrium increases further in thickness, and accumulation of water continues. The glands become enormously dilated, present a saw-tooth appearance in section, and produce a secretion, rich in mucin and glycogen, termed *uterine milk*. The stroma cells of the strata compactum and spongiosum enlarge, become polyhedral and accumulate glycogen and lipids in the *predecidual reaction*. The spiral arteries enlarge slightly and become tightly coiled. The venous network becomes even more complex and shows large dilatations. Direct arteriovenous anastomoses are a prominent feature at this stage.

If fertilization and implantation take place, hCG keeps the corpus luteum secreting oestrogens and progesterone, the progestational phase continues and menstruation does not occur. If fertilization fails to occur, the corpus luteum is not maintained and the oestrogen and progesterone levels fall. The progestational endometrium is thus deprived of the hormonal stimulus which maintains it, and retrogresses. The endometrium loses fluid and decreases in thickness as the stromal cells shrink and the glands buckle. The spiral vessels are thus compressed and their bases undergo intermittent constriction and relaxation. This results in venous stasis and patchy ischaemic necrosis in the superficial tissues. Rupture of damaged vessel walls follows, causing subepithelial haemorrhages which further disrupt the tissues. Continuation of this process leads to haemorrhage into the uterine cavity and piecemeal shedding of the tissues of the strata compactum and spongiosum as the *menses*. The stratum basale and the short straight arteries remain unchanged throughout the menstrual cycle. Regeneration of the epithelium occurs from the torn bases of the glands in the stratum basale, and a new proliferative phase is entered.

Menstruation at puberty, near the menopause and, occasionally, at other times may follow an *anovulatory* cycle. In the absence of progesterone the endometrium may be shed in patches with excessive bleeding if the stimulus of oestrogen continues or as a whole if the stimulus is withdrawn.

In most mammals reproductive life is divided into a number of breeding or sexual seasons. During each season there are one or more times when the female is on heat (i.e. is receptive of the male). This phenomenon is called *oestrus*. At the beginning of a sexual season the gonads and genital tract are quiescent but they soon enter a phase of activity—*pro-oestrus*—in which growth of ovarian follicles and increased oestrogen production leads to congestion of the whole genital tract and proliferation and oedema of the endometrium. This culminates in an *oestrus* phase, during which ovulation occurs. At this stage there may be some bleeding from the hyperaemic proliferative endometrium. If mating does not occur the generative organs become quiescent. A longer (*anoestrus*) or shorter (*dioestrus*) period of quiescence follows and leads into another oestrus cycle. Successful mating is followed by a period of gestation, which ends with parturition, and then a recovery period during which nursing or lactation takes place. The time interval between parturition and the onset of

The Female Reproductive Cycles

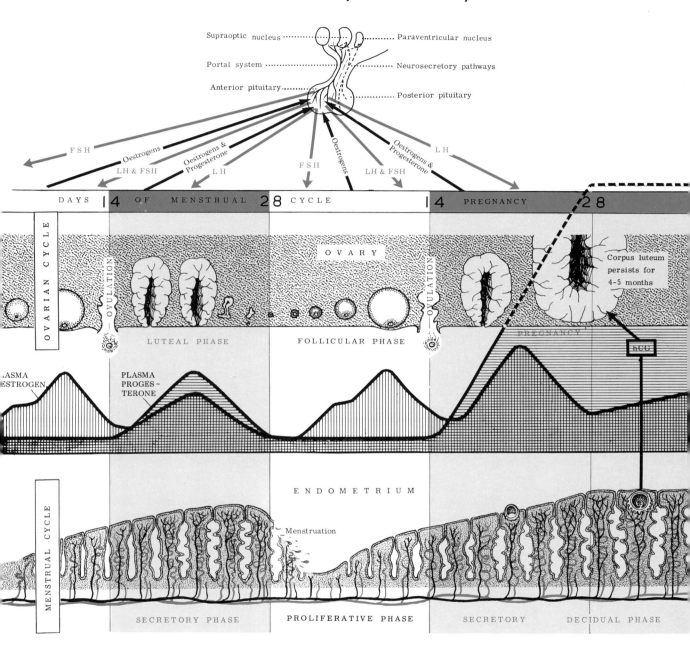

another oestrus cycle is extremely variable. In some mammals, particularly if sterile mating has occurred, oestrus is followed by a period of pseudo-pregnancy. This consists of a secretory reaction of the endometrium in response to progesterone secreted by a corpus luteum of pseudo-pregnancy. With regression of the corpus luteum the pseudo-pregnant endometrium gradually degenerates and an anoestrus or dioestrus phase is entered. Sometimes the degeneration of a pseudo-pregnant endometrium is accompanied by slight uterine haemorrhage.

The oestrus bleeding which occurs in some mammals does not correspond to the menstrual flux of the human female, but may correspond more closely to the slight blood-stained discharge—the *Kleine Regel*—which some women have at mid-cycle. This discharge, from a proliferative endometrium near ovulation time, may be accompanied by low abdominal pain—the *Mittelschmerz*. Human menstruation may thus be regarded as the haemorrhagic degeneration of a pseudo-pregnant endometrium.

Mammals may be classified according to the number of ova they normally shed at ovulation. The offspring of *polyovulatory* species (e.g. cat) are termed litter mates. The term 'fraternal twins' is limited to the non-identical offspring of species which are normally *monovulatory* (e.g. man) or *diovulatory* (e.g. marmoset). Thus, in man, *fraternal (dizygotic) twins* follow the fertilization of two ova. Such twins are as genetically dissimilar as other members of the same family, but may show secondary fusion of their extraembryonic membranes. *Polyembryonic* or *identical (monozygotic) twins* develop from a single fertilized ovum. They are thus of the same sex, resemble each other closely and are genetically identical. An inherited form of polyembryony is the rule in certain species of armadillo, occurs occasionally in man, and may infrequently be associated with anomalies of development. A sporadic non-inherited form occurs uncommonly in all species, including man, and, in addition to identical twins, may result in various forms of double monster.

The stage at which separation of embryonic material occurs varies. Identical twins can be produced in amphibia by the separation of the blastomeres at the two-celled stage. In man it is more likely that separation occurs at the inner cell mass stage. For twins to be produced the plane of separation must necessarily transect the area containing future presumptive chorda-mesoderm. The membrane relationships of identical twins vary with the stage of separation (p. 62).

Before puberty the human female reproductive tract is immature, with little or no pituitary gonadotrophic or ovarian hormones being produced. *Puberty* is the period during which the genital tract matures and the secondary sexual characteristics develop. It ends with the first menstrual period—the *menarche*. During puberty the output of gonadotrophins rises and the ovaries are stimulated to produce the oestrogens which cause the maturation changes. The menarche commonly occurs between the ages of 12 and 15 but may be somewhat earlier or later without pathological significance. In the first 2 or 3 years after the menarche, menstrual irregularities are common and include prolonged cycle and missed periods—*amenorrhoea*. During this period of adolescent sterility, the majority of ovarian cycles are probably anovulatory, and full reproductive capacity—*nubility*—with regular ovulatory cycles is not achieved. Thereafter, ovulatory cycles normally continue, except in pregnancy, until the *climacteric*.

Conception may follow coitus at any time but is most likely to follow insemination near mid-cycle (ovulation). A period of gestation follows, during which the developing embryo is carried in the gravid uterus. The human gestation period is about 266 days. It ends at term with the full development of the conceptus and the onset of labour or parturition. Labour consists of the successive expulsion of the fetus and afterbirth (placenta, extraembryonic membranes and a part of the uterine lining). During the puerperium, which follows, the genital tract involutes and lactation is established. Ovulation and menstruation do not often begin again during lactation but pregnancy sometimes follows fertilization of the first ovum to be shed after delivery—i.e. before menstruation is re-established. A woman who has not borne a child is termed a *nullipara*; one who has borne children is termed a *multipara*.

The *climacteric* is a period of gradual reduction in the cyclic activity of the ovaries, and culminates when menstruation ceases at the *menopause*. At the climacteric, cycles may increase in length, the menses become increasingly scanty or menstruation may cease abruptly without either of these changes. Anovulatory cycles not infrequently occur. After the menopause the production of ovarian hormones ceases and the uterus, vagina and mammary glands become atrophic. The level of circulating gonadotrophin, however, continues to rise to a peak value 15–20 years after the menopause.

Age and the Uterus

NEWBORN   NULLIPARA   MULTIPARA   SENESCENT

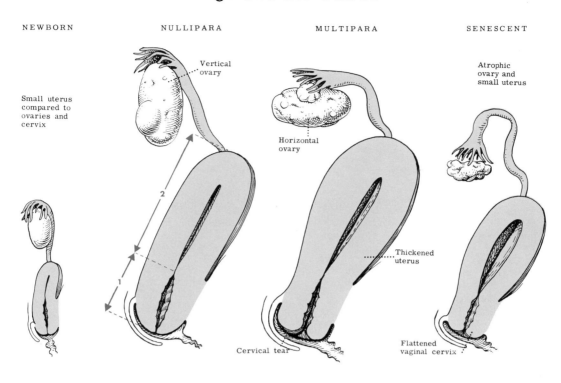

Small uterus compared to ovaries and cervix

Vertical ovary

Horizontal ovary

Atrophic ovary and small uterus

Thickened uterus

Cervical tear

Flattened vaginal cervix

Pregnancy and the Uterus

CONTOUR OF THE GRAVID UTERUS AT DIFFERENT STAGES OF PREGNANCY

FULL-TERM GRAVID UTERUS
note disposition of the uterine tubes, round ligaments and ovaries

POSTPARTUM CONTOURS OF THE INVOLUTING UTERUS

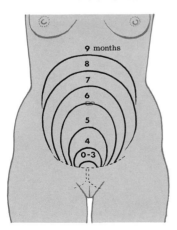

9 months
8
7
6
5
4
0-3

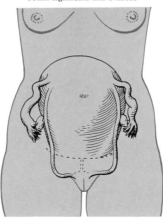

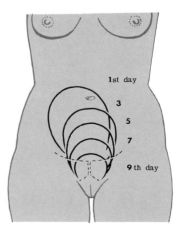

1st day
3
5
7
9 th day

Fertilization and implantation

At ovulation the *secondary oocyte*, with an eccentrically placed *second maturation spindle*, is surrounded by its plasma membrane outside which lies the *first polar body*. The oocyte and polar body are enclosed in the *zona pellucida*, which is covered by the cells of the *corona radiata* making up the *cumulus oophorus*. The fimbriated end of the uterine tube becomes closely applied to, and partially covers, the ovary, so that the oocyte is swept into the uterine tube. In the absence of fertilization the oocyte is carried down the tube by fluid currents generated by ciliary action and irregular peristaltic waves. It becomes non-viable within a day or two.

Sperms enter the cervical canal, become aligned on cervical mucus strands and pass up through the cavity of the uterus to the uterine tube. This they do as a result of contractions of the uterus and countercurrent flow in the tube together with active swimming movements. They reach the ampullary end of the tube in minutes rather than hours, and they attain and retain their fertilizing power for 2–3 days. *Fertilization* normally occurs in the outer third of the uterine tube. The oocyte and its coverings have no specific attracting force for the sperms and only random contacts are made. As sperms approach the oocyte, the superficial part of the acrosomal cap dissolves: hyaluronidase and acrosin are released and the deeper part is exposed. The *hyaluronidase* causes separation and falling away of the cells of the corona radiata, and *acrosin*—a proteolytic enzyme—facilitates penetration of the zona pellucida. When a sperm reaches the surface of the oocyte the postacrosomal region of the head adheres to it and their membranes fuse; the sperm is then enveloped by cytoplasm and the oocyte is *activated*. Initially this involves complex changes in the oocyte surface, which reduce the possibility of further sperm entry or *polyspermy*: cortical granules fuse with the cell membrane and release their contents into the *perivitelline space*; this normally prevents further sperm entry. The second maturation spindle now completes its division with the extrusion of a second polar body and the formation of an eccentrically placed female pronucleus. The head of the engulfed sperm swells, forming a male pronucleus and centrioles, other parts degenerate. The pronuclei and centrioles migrate towards the centre of the cell and engage in *syngamy*:

the centrioles separate and form a cleavage spindle, the nuclear membranes of the pronuclei disappear and their chromosomes, the DNA of which has already replicated, become arranged around its equator. The first cleavage division follows.

Fertilization thus results in a restoration of the diploid number of chromosomes, the determination of the chromosomal sex of the new individual and the initiation of cleavage. The polarity of the oocyte and the site of sperm entry probably effectively determine regional cytoplasmic differences in the zygote which are important in subsequent developmental mechanisms.

A series of cleavage divisions results in a mulberry-shaped mass of blastomeres—the *morula*—surrounded by the zona pellucida. This occurs during the 3–4 days taken for passage through the uterine tube, which is effected by ciliary action and peristalsis. During the next 3–4 days, while free in the uterine cavity, the morula develops into a *blastocyst* within the zona pellucida. The cellular wall of the blastocyst comprises the first extraembryonic membrane, the blastocystic or primary *trophoblast*. Before about the seventh day after fertilization the blastocyst escapes from the zona pellucida and the exposed cells of the trophoblast attach to the surface of the endometrium, usually between the mouths of uterine glands. The adhering region of the trophoblast overlies the inner cell mass and differentiates into two primitive layers. An inner germinative layer of cells, the *cytotrophoblast*, adds to an outer syncytial layer, the *syncytiotrophoblast*. The latter has active invasive properties and erodes maternal epithelia, stroma and blood vessels to form a ragged *implantation cavity* into which the blastocyst sinks (*interstitial implantation*). At the time of implantation the endometrium is at the height of the secretory phase. After implantation it is called the *decidua*, and *capsular*, *basal* and *parietal zones* are recognized. Throughout the early months of pregnancy the decidua retains the structural characteristics of the secretory phase in exaggerated form. The stromal cells increase further in size, become vacuolated and accumulate additional glycogen, lipids and mitochondria as they become *decidual cells*. The walls of the implantation cavity and the trophoblast are concerned in the development of the placenta.

Within 24 hours of fertilization an immunosuppressive protein—*early pregnancy factor* (EPF)—appears in maternal serum. EPF may thus form the basis of a test for pregnancy prior to implantation.

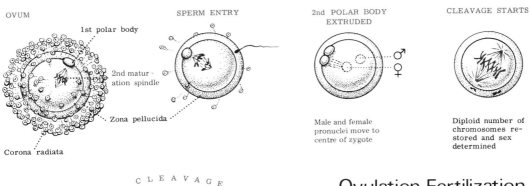

OVUM

1st polar body

2nd maturation spindle

Zona pellucida

Corona radiata

SPERM ENTRY

2nd POLAR BODY EXTRUDED

Male and female pronuclei move to centre of zygote

CLEAVAGE STARTS

Diploid number of chromosomes restored and sex determined

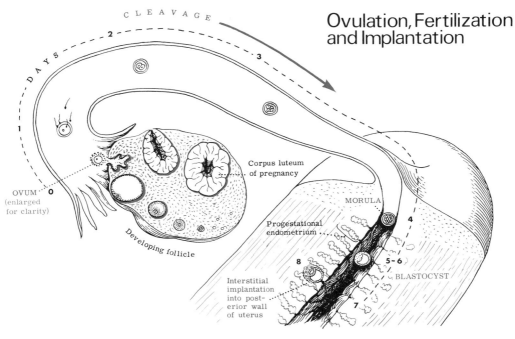

Ovulation, Fertilization and Implantation

CLEAVAGE

DAYS

1

2

3

4

OVUM (enlarged for clarity)

0

Developing follicle

Corpus luteum of pregnancy

Progestational endometrium

MORULA

5-6

BLASTOCYST

8

7

Interstitial implantation into posterior wall of uterus

The Gravid Uterus

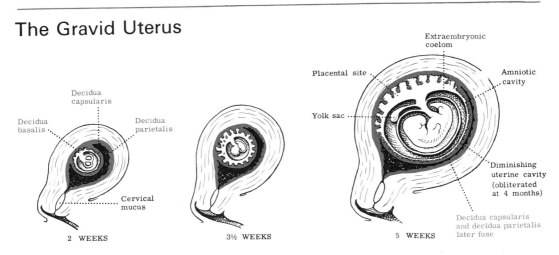

Decidua capsularis

Decidua basalis

Decidua parietalis

Cervical mucus

2 WEEKS

3½ WEEKS

Placental site

Yolk sac

Extraembryonic coelom

Amniotic cavity

Diminishing uterine cavity (obliterated at 4 months)

Decidua capsularis and decidua parietalis later fuse

5 WEEKS

The Embryo, Placenta and Membranes

In the second week the embryo consists of a two-layered disc between two cavities, the whole being suspended by a *connecting stalk* within a third cavity. These fluid-filled cavities are important because they bring nutrients into direct contact with the cells of the embryo and facilitate their movement. The loose connective tissue lining the *extraembryonic coelom* (Gk = cavity) is called *mesoderm*; with the trophoblast, it forms the membrane called the *chorion* which nutrients and fluid must cross to pass in from the implantation cavity. With cells lining the *amniotic* and *yolk cavities*, mesoderm forms the membranes called the *amnion* and the *yolk sac* which also must be crossed to reach the embryo. An outgrowth from the yolk sac forms the membrane called the *allantois* which grows into the connecting stalk where it produces cells which form blood vessels. Later the allantois forms a temporary receptacle for fetal urine. Of these *extraembryonic membranes* the yolk sac is present in fishes such as the shark but the others are adaptations to terrestrial life and reproduce in miniature the total aquatic environment in which ancestral forms evolved.

Cells from the floor of the amniotic cavity turn in and spread between the two layers of the embryonic disc, creating a third layer. The *ectoderm* (outer skin) will form the epithelium on the surface of the body and organs which develop by ingrowth from it, the *endoderm* (inner skin) the lining of the gut and organs which develop by outgrowths from it, while the *mesoderm* (middle skin) will form organs and most connective tissues between them. Occupying the midline in the middle layer (hence called *chorda-mesoderm*) is the *notochord*, a rod of cells which gives the embryo some rigidity. Although only vestiges of the notochord persist, it places man squarely in the phylum Chordata.

In front of and behind the notochord, ectoderm and endoderm remain in contact at the *oral membrane* and the *cloacal membrane*. Under the influence of the underlying chorda-mesoderm the ectoderm between these membranes thickens and forms the *neural plate*, the side lips of which fold up into the amniotic cavity and meet in the midline to form the *neural tube*. At first the tube has open ends but these close and it forms the early spinal cord and brain.

The amniotic cavity expands around the embryonic disc, the edges of which grow round and enclose *head, tail* and *lateral embryonic folds*. In this process part of the yolk cavity becomes included within the embryo as the *primitive gut*, the *foregut* extending forwards to the oral membrane, the *midgut* lying over the remaining part of the yolk sac and the *hindgut* extending backwards to the cloacal membrane. The expanding amniotic cavity and the edges of the disc then converge at the *umbilicus*, which encloses the connecting stalk and a narrow duct leading from the midgut to the yolk sac. Thus the *umbilical cord* is covered in amnion and leads from the embryo to the chorion.

The body of the embryo is now too large and complex for its cells to exchange gases, nutrients and waste materials directly with surrounding cavities. Instead, there develops a vascular system to transport fluids, via the umbilical cord, between the tissues of the embryo and the placenta, an organ specialized for exchanges between fetal and maternal bloods. The chorion extends finger-like processes (*villi*) into the *decidua basalis* so that the surface area for absorption from the implantation cavity is increased. Later, villi extend into the *decidua capsularis* all around the conceptus. Later still, villi again become limited to the decidua basalis, the site of the definitive placenta. In the placenta, fetal and maternal bloods remain separated by the tissue of the chorionic villi which generally acts as a *placental barrier* to infection of the fetus by the mother but permits the exchange of metabolites. The chorion initially secretes hormones which stimulate the ovary so that the corpus luteum persists and continues to secrete the oestrogens and progesterone necessary for the continuation of pregnancy. Later the placenta itself produces these and other hormones and the corpus luteum atrophies.

The placenta performs the respiratory functions of the lungs and many of the metabolic functions of the liver for the fetus, so these organs only become fully functional after birth. Once the baby is born the placenta is redundant and is delivered with the membranes as the afterbirth.

Embryogenesis

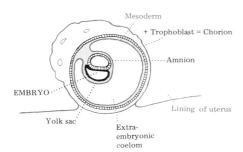

Mesoderm
+ Trophoblast = Chorion
Amnion
EMBRYO
Lining of uterus
Yolk sac
Extra-embryonic coelom

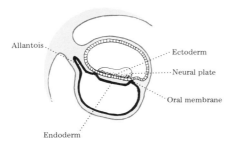

Allantois
Ectoderm
Neural plate
Oral membrane
Endoderm

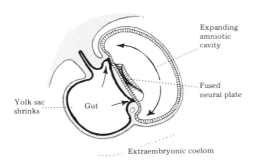

Expanding amniotic cavity
Fused neural plate
Yolk sac shrinks
Gut
Extraembryonic coelom

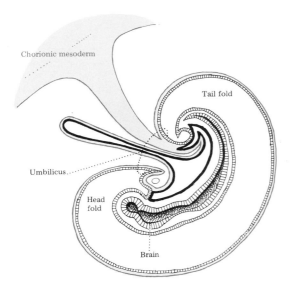

Chorionic mesoderm
Tail fold
Umbilicus
Head fold
Brain

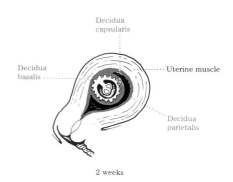

Decidua capsularis
Decidua basalis
Uterine muscle
Decidua parietalis

2 weeks

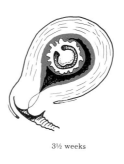

3½ weeks

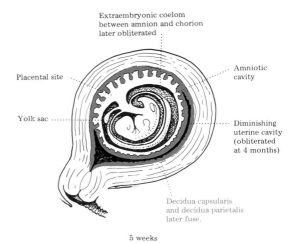

Extraembryonic coelom between amnion and chorion later obliterated
Placental site
Amniotic cavity
Yolk sac
Diminishing uterine cavity (obliterated at 4 months)
Decidua capsularis and decidua parietalis later fuse.

5 weeks

Cleavage and blastocyst formation

At the time of fertilization the oocyte is atypical, compared with general somatic cells, in that it has an enormous cytoplasmic/nuclear ratio. Cleavage involves a series of rapid mitotic divisions with synthesis of DNA, but no increase in cytoplasmic mass and therefore a return to the usual cytoplasmic/nuclear ratio. The resulting blastomeres are small, which facilitates morphogenetic movements, and, as the cytoplasm of the oocyte has regional differences, they have differing nucleocytoplasmic relationships.

The first cleavage division results in two blastomeres of equal size. Cleavage remains regular and distinct until the 8-cell stage when the cells become polyhedral and fit together (*compaction*), permitting the formation of gap and tight junctions between them. Thereafter cleavage is less regular and the *morula* of 16–32 cells is made up of inside cells and outside cells, only the latter having tight junctions between them.

Fluid-filled spaces appear between the inside cells of the morula and soon coalesce to form a *blastocystic cavity*. As in other similar situations, the origin of the fluid has been ascribed to the activity of a sodium pump, to endosmosis of fluid from outside, to secretion by surrounding cells or to central cellular degeneration. The outside cells of the resulting *blastocyst* make up the *trophoblast* and now have tight, gap and adhering junctions between them. Inside the trophoblast is the blastocystic cavity and an eccentrically placed *inner cell mass*. The area of contact between the inner cell mass and the overlying polar trophoblast defines the *embryonic pole* of the blastocyst. After the blastocyst escapes from the zona pellucida, the polar trophoblast attaches to the endometrium and differentiates into syncytiotrophoblast and cytotrophoblast. As implantation proceeds, the formation of these two trophoblastic layers continues around the blastocyst and eventually reaches the *abembryonic pole*. There, the syncytial layer remains much thinner than at the embryonic pole.

Meanwhile the inner cell mass differentiates into a layer of cuboidal cells—*the hypoblast*—bordering the blastocystic cavity and a mass of cells—*the epiblast*—between the hypoblast and the polar trophoblast. The cells of the epiblast and hypoblast are *epithelial*—that is, they comprise compact ordered sheets or masses of cells; the epiblast and hypoblast are, however, separated by a basement membrane. Cells which differentiate from the edge of the hypoblast and spread inside the trophoblast to enclose a *primary yolk cavity* are *mesenchymatous*—that is, they are loosely arranged stellate cells. Having enclosed the primary yolk cavity, mesenchymatous cells then form a fenestrated lining for it and a reticulum between the lining and the trophoblast.

While these changes have been occurring, a *primary amniotic cavity* has developed in the epiblast close to the trophoblast. Its thin epiblastic roof breaks down so that a transient *trophoepiblastic cavity* with a floor of stratified columnar epiblastic cells is formed. From the edge of the epiblast rather flatter *amniogenic cells* spread to line the *secondary amniotic cavity* (cf. fold formation in other amniotes, p. 30). The yolk and amniotic cavities permit morphogenetic movements of the cells of the embryonic disc.

Meanwhile the first signs of the craniocaudal axis of the embryo appear: a thickening of the hypoblast at the anterior end forms the *prechordal plate*, and a loosening of the epiblast at the posterior end forms the *primitive streak*; both are precocious compared with their non-human homologues. The prechordal plate develops specific adhesiveness to overlying epiblast and, by proliferation, later becomes a source of head mesenchyme. The primitive streak is a site of morphogenetic movements and cells stream from its ventral aspect. Initially they pass laterally and caudodorsally to form a layer of *extraembryonic mesoderm* between the amniogenic (*extraembryonic ectoderm*) cells and trophoblast.

Again, while these changes have been occurring the distal part of the primary yolk sac has collapsed and fragmented; its proximal part forms the *secondary yolk sac* and the cells lining it become epithelial *extraembryonic endoderm*. Extraembryonic mesoderm from the primitive streak streams ventrally outside the mesenchymatous reticulum to line the trophoblast and outside the endoderm of the secondary yolk sac to envelop it. With the degeneration of the reticulum and the remnants of the primary yolk sac there develops an *extraembryonic coelom* which is completely lined with extraembryonic mesoderm. The extraembryonic coelom soon extends dorsally into the extraembryonic mesoderm between the amniotic ectoderm and the trophoblast except at one point where a mesodermal strand—the *connecting stalk*—remains between the polar trophoblast and the posterior end of the embryo. A small diverticulum from the hypoblast—the *allantois*—grows into the connecting stalk and contributes precocious allantoic mesenchyme to it. With the development of the extraembryonic coelom, the extraembryonic mesoderm has been divided into two zones—*somatopleuric* in contact with amniogenic cells or with trophoblast, and *splanchnopleuric* in contact with endoderm. The early extraembryonic membranes—*amnion, chorion, yolk sac* and *allantois*—can now be recognized.

Cleavage and Implantation

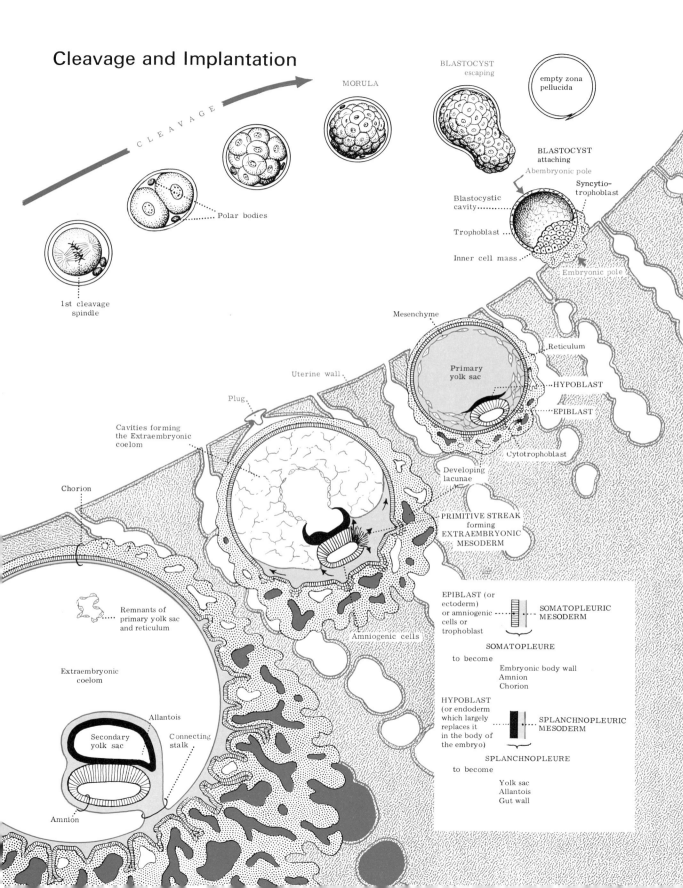

CLEAVAGE

MORULA

BLASTOCYST
escaping

empty zona
pellucida

Polar bodies

1st cleavage
spindle

BLASTOCYST
attaching

Abembryonic pole

Syncytio-
trophoblast

Blastocystic
cavity

Trophoblast

Inner cell mass

Embryonic pole

Mesenchyme

Uterine wall

Plug

Reticulum

Primary
yolk sac

HYPOBLAST

EPIBLAST

Cavities forming
the Extraembryonic
coelom

Cytotrophoblast

Developing
lacunae

Chorion

PRIMITIVE STREAK
forming
EXTRAEMBRYONIC
MESODERM

Remnants of
primary yolk sac
and reticulum

Amniogenic cells

Extraembryonic
coelom

EPIBLAST (or
ectoderm)
or amniogenic
cells or
trophoblast

SOMATOPLEURIC
MESODERM

SOMATOPLEURE

to become

Embryonic body wall
Amnion
Chorion

Allantois

Secondary
yolk sac

Connecting
stalk

HYPOBLAST
(or endoderm
which largely
replaces it
in the body of
the embryo)

SPLANCHNOPLEURIC
MESODERM

SPLANCHNOPLEURE

to become

Yolk sac
Allantois
Gut wall

Amnion

Embryogenesis

Soon after implantation the *bilaminar embryonic disc* is approximately circular in outline. There is a zone of mesoderm at the margin of the disc, between epiblast and hypoblast as they diverge to become continuous with the ectodermal and endodermal linings of the amniotic and yolk sac cavities respectively. This *junctional zone* lies between the somatopleuric mesoderm of the amnion and the splanchnopleuric mesoderm of the yolk sac. With extension of the extraembryonic coelom the connecting stalk becomes restricted to the posterior edge of the disc where it is continuous with the junctional zone of mesoderm. The anterior part of the junctional zone is called the *septum transversum*.

The features of the midline are thus the septum transversum and the prechordal plate anteriorly and the primitive streak and connecting stalk posteriorly. The primitive streak is now seen as a distinct linear opacity in the epiblast. The opacity is due to cell accumulation and morphogenetic movement as cells from the epiblast stream through the primitive streak. The first cells to do so form extraembryonic mesoderm; later cells form intraembryonic mesoderm and endoderm. Embryonic mesoderm streams between the two layers of the embryonic disc, making it trilaminar and forming the embryonic mesoderm; cells from the primitive streak probably replace the hypoblast in the roof of the secondary yolk sac and form embryonic endoderm. The epiblastic cells which remain on the surface constitute the embryonic ectoderm.

A locus of cell proliferation—the *primitive node*—is found at the anterior tip of the primitive streak, between it and the posterior edge of the prechordal plate. Cells from the primitive node spread anteriorly and laterally as ectoderm; some pass posteriorly through the primitive streak while yet others pass anteriorly from the under-surface of the node as the *notochordal process*. This solid column of cells tracks forwards between ectoderm and endoderm in the axial plane and appears to push the posterior edge of the prechordal plate ahead of it. As mesoderm cells continue to flow from the primitive streak, and the notochordal process continues to lengthen, the embryonic disc becomes elongated and pear-shaped. Beginning at the primitive node, a notochordal canal (continuous with the amniotic cavity) develops throughout the notochordal process. The ventral wall of the canal fuses with the endodermal roof of the yolk sac and then breaks down, establishing a communication between the amniotic and yolk sac cavities. The dorsal wall of the notochordal canal thus forms an axial strip—the *notochordal plate*—in the roof

of the yolk sac (cf. the amphibian archenteron). Beginning anteriorly the notochordal plate then folds off to form an axial solid column of cells—the definitive *notochord*—and the roof of the yolk sac is reconstituted, probably by embryonic endoderm of primitive streak origin. The processes of fusion, breakdown and reconstitution begin cranially and proceed caudally so that, for a while, a canal connecting the amniotic and yolk sac cavities persists caudally. As the neural groove develops, this canal transiently connects its hind end with the lumen of the primitive gut (cf. the amphibian neurenteric canal).

Meanwhile the primitive streak appears to move forwards and, as the *allantois* grows into the connecting stalk, the endoderm of the hind end of the roof of the yolk sac comes into intimate apposition with overlying ectoderm to form the *cloacal membrane* (structures may now be homologized with the amphibian blastopore *seriatim*: the primitive node with the dorsal lip, the primitive streak with the fused lateral lips and the region of the cloacal membrane with the ventral lip). Correspondingly, near the anterior edge of the embryonic disc is another area of endodermal/ectodermal adhesion which includes part of the prechordal plate and its overlying ectoderm, and which forms the *oral membrane*.

Except at the oral and cloacal membranes, ectoderm and endoderm become separated by the third layer of the embryonic disc—the *chorda-mesoderm* (notochord and mesoderm). While the notochord grows from the primitive node, mesodermal cells flow from the primitive streak and spread between ectoderm and endoderm, anteriorly, laterally and posteriorly, as bilateral sheets. Each mesodermal sheet passes forwards, alongside the notochord, and skirts the margins of the oral membrane to meet the sheet of the opposite side as the cardiogenic area of mesoderm. This lies immediately anterior to the oral membrane and merges with the mesoderm of the septum transversum. Each sheet spreads laterally, separating ectoderm and endoderm, to meet and merge with the junctional zone of extraembryonic mesoderm. From the posterior end of the primitive streak, each sheet spreads round the margins of the cloacal membrane to merge with, and contribute to, the mesoderm of the connecting stalk.

Epiblast has thus formed embryonic ectoderm, chorda-mesoderm and endoderm, the extraembryonic ectoderm of the amnion and the extraembryonic mesoderm of the chorion, amnion and yolk sac. *Hypoblast* has probably formed only the embryonic endoderm of the prechordal plate and cloacal membrane and the extraembryonic endoderm of the yolk sac and allantois.

Early Embryogenesis

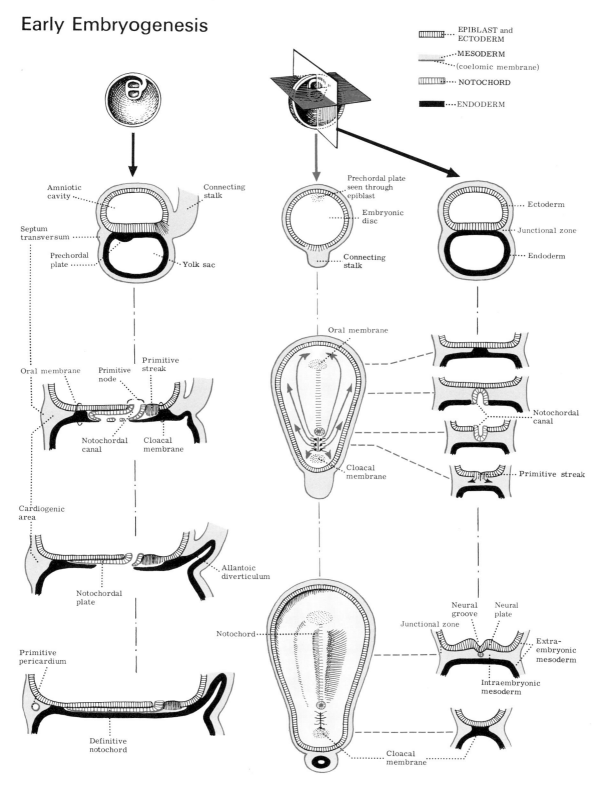

EPIBLAST and ECTODERM

MESODERM
(coelomic membrane)

NOTOCHORD

ENDODERM

Amniotic cavity

Connecting stalk

Septum transversum

Prechordal plate

Yolk sac

Prechordal plate seen through epiblast

Embryonic disc

Connecting stalk

Ectoderm

Junctional zone

Endoderm

Oral membrane

Primitive node

Primitive streak

Notochordal canal

Cloacal membrane

Oral membrane

Notochordal canal

Primitive streak

Cloacal membrane

Cardiogenic area

Notochordal plate

Allantoic diverticulum

Primitive pericardium

Definitive notochord

Notochord

Junctional zone

Neural groove

Neural plate

Extra-embryonic mesoderm

Intraembryonic mesoderm

Cloacal membrane

The early trilaminar embryo has the form of a somewhat flattened pear-shaped plate. Subsequent changes of shape are dominated by the formation and growth of the neural tube, the regional differentiation of the intraembryonic mesoderm, the appearance of an intraembryonic coelom and the expansion of the amnion.

Under the influence of underlying chorda-mesoderm, the axial strip of ectoderm between the primitive node and the oral membrane thickens to form the *neural plate*. The plate is wider anteriorly and soon develops a longitudinal *neural groove*. It is surrounded peripherally by a ridge of *presumptive neural crest* tissue (p. 125). As the groove deepens, the lateral margins of the plate become raised and turned in so that they fuse near their mid-point and form the *neural tube*. Ectoderm becomes continuous across the dorsal aspect of the tube. Neural tube formation then proceeds cranially and caudally but the extremities of the tube remain open for a while at the *anterior* and *posterior neuropores*. Cranially the neural plate shows three expansions which, after closure, form three *primary brain vesicles*. The neural tube grows rapidly in length, develops a dorsal curvature and soon begins to bulge upwards into the amniotic cavity.

Meanwhile the intraembryonic mesoderm has differentiated into three main regions: a *paraxial* strip flanks the notochord; an *intermediate* strip lies lateral to this; and a *lateral plate* extends from the edge of the intermediate mesoderm to the junctional zone of extraembryonic mesoderm. Beginning cranially and extending caudally, the *paraxial mesoderm* becomes segmented (metameric segmentation) into a series of blocks—the *somites*. Each somite contributes to two adjacent vertebrae and their intervertebral disc, to a segmental mass of somatic muscle and to the overlying dermis. The *intermediate mesoderm* contributes to the kidney system, the gonads and the suprarenal glands.

The sheets of *lateral plate mesoderm*, which are continuous with each other at the cardiogenic area, develop multiple clefts which coalesce and form an intraembryonic coelom. At first, this single horseshoe-shaped cavity is closed. Each limb lies in the lateral plate alongside the intermediate mesoderm. The connecting loop, which lies in the cardiogenic area, forms the primitive pericardial cavity. Lateral plate mesoderm is thus divided into two layers which bound the coelom. Somatopleuric mesoderm is in contact with ectoderm, and splanchnopleuric mesoderm is in contact with endoderm. Initially the lateral wall of each coelomic limb is formed by the junctional zone of extraembryonic mesoderm, but soon this breaks down in its caudal half and a communication is established between the intraembryonic and the extraembryonic coelom. The communication is co-extensive with the future midgut which has, therefore, no ventral mesentery.

The rapid growth of the nervous system and the expansion of the amniotic cavity result in important changes in relative position of the principal derivatives of the disc. The forebrain bulges upwards and forwards into the amniotic cavity, and the septum transversum, pericardium and oral membrane swing on to its ventral surface. Eventually they undergo a complete reversal of position. The septum transversum, initially anterior to the pericardium, becomes ventral and, finally, posterior to it. Similarly, at the hind end of the embryo, the attachment of the connecting stalk with its contained allantois passes progressively onto the ventral surface. These processes of head- and tail-fold formation, together with less pronounced lateral folding, result in the inclusion of the upper part of the secondary yolk cavity within the embryonic body as the primitive gut. Tail-fold formation also draws the coelom between the allantois and yolk sac into the body so that the hindgut has no ventral mesentery.

With continued expansion of the amnion, its line of embryonic attachment becomes a decreasing ellipse on the ventral body wall—the *primitive umbilicus*. The *umbilical cord* is thus covered externally by amniotic somatopleure, which encloses the connecting stalk (and allantois), the splanchnopleure of the narrowing stalk (vitellointestinal duct) of the yolk sac and the communication between the intraembryonic and the extraembryonic coelomic cavities.

The *midgut* lies over the narrowing yolk sac. The *foregut* extends anteriorly to the oral membrane and lies dorsal to the roof of the primitive pericardial cavity and the septum transversum. The *hindgut* extends posteriorly to the cloacal membrane and the endodermal allantois leads from its ventral wall; a small recess—the *postanal gut*—continues into the tail.

With advancing head-, tail- and lateral-fold formation the simple pear-shaped embryonic disc gradually assumes a recognizable comma-shaped embryonic form with a cranial dilatation and a gently curving trunk and tail. This primary embryonic curve, convex dorsally, is reflected in the form of all the early longitudinal structures, including the neural tube, notochord, primitive gut, paraxial and intermediate mesoderm, and in the caudally directed limbs of the intraembryonic coelom. Soon, however, the curve is complicated cranially by the appearance of three flexures affecting the early nervous system. A *cervical flexure* and a *midbrain flexure* are convex dorsally and an *intermediate (pontine) flexure* is convex ventrally.

Head, Tail and Lateral Folds

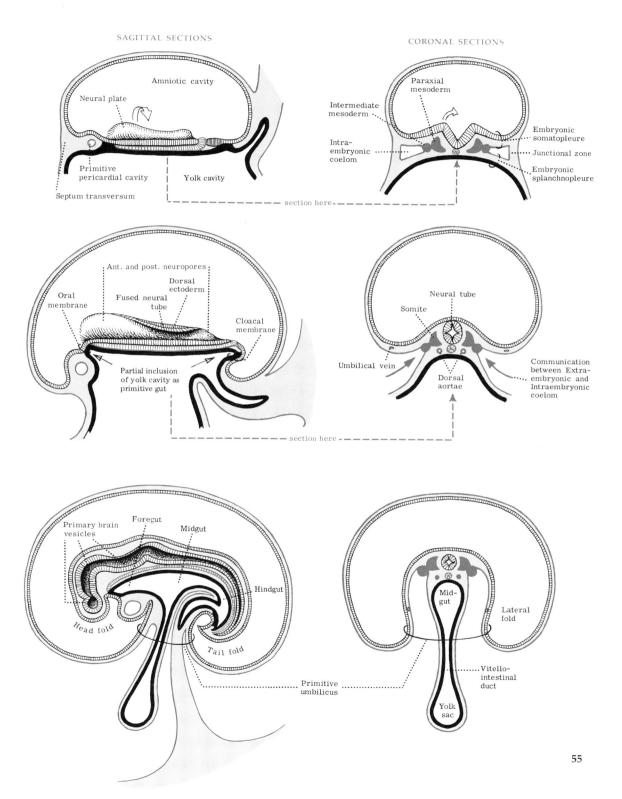

SAGITTAL SECTIONS

CORONAL SECTIONS

Amniotic cavity

Neural plate

Primitive pericardial cavity

Yolk cavity

Septum transversum

Paraxial mesoderm

Intermediate mesoderm

Intra-embryonic coelom

Embryonic somatopleure

Junctional zone

Embryonic splanchnopleure

section here

Ant. and post. neuropores

Dorsal ectoderm

Fused neural tube

Oral membrane

Cloacal membrane

Partial inclusion of yolk cavity as primitive gut

Neural tube

Somite

Umbilical vein

Dorsal aortae

Communication between Extra-embryonic and Intraembryonic coelom

section here

Primary brain vesicles

Foregut

Midgut

Hindgut

Head fold

Tail fold

Primitive umbilicus

Mid-gut

Lateral fold

Vitello-intestinal duct

Yolk sac

The ventral aspect of an embryo thus shows, in series from the cranial end: a highly convex swelling caused by the underlying forebrain vesicle; the oral membrane lying in the floor of an ectodermal pit, the *stomodeum*; a large convex pericardial swelling; the decreasing ellipse of the primitive umbilicus; the oval depression of the cloacal membrane; and, finally, the ventral surface of the tail.

The *amnion* remains important in subsequent development. With the expansion of the amniotic cavity, the extraembryonic coelom is obliterated, except in the proximal part of the umbilical cord, and the amnion and chorion fuse. The *liquor amnii* provides a medium in which the embryo and fetus can develop and move freely. In the first half of pregnancy similarities in composition with fetal body fluids suggest that it is a transudate. In the second half, however, the fetus swallows large quantities of liquor and returns fluid to the cavity as urine and as lung secretions, some of which are immediately swallowed. About 1 litre at term, its volume may be more (*hydramnios*) or less (*oligohydramnios*) than normal depending upon disturbance of the circulating mechanisms, upon fetal abnormalities (of which *anencephaly* is by far the commonest cause of hydramnios), upon maternal conditions and upon unknown factors. The amniotic cavity may be tapped (*amniocentesis*), making possible the diagnosis of some fetal conditions in utero.

Two principal types of tissues are present in the embryo—epithelial and mesenchymatous.

Epithelial tissues are essentially ordered sheets of cells, with little intercellular substance, bounding the surfaces and lining the various body cavities of the embryo; they have specialized juxtaluminal junctions and develop basement membranes. Such tissues include the primitive ectoderm and most of its derivatives, including the early neural plate and the primitive endoderm and most of its derivatives. They also include the linings of cavities and duct systems which develop from mesoderm: the epithelia lining the coelomic cavity, the synovial cavities, the blood vascular and lymphatic systems, the gonads, kidneys and their ducts, and the walls of transient cavities in the somites.

Mesenchymatous tissues consist of loosely arranged stellate cells suspended in a gelatinous matrix; they are linked only by tight and gap junctions. The cells are amoeboid and actively phagocytic, and their processes make temporary contact with those of overlying epithelial cells and their basement membranes as they migrate. Such tissues are largely mesodermal in origin but may be derived from the other germ layers; e.g. the ectoderm of the neural crest and of various placodes together with the endoderm of the prechordal plate contribute to head mesenchyme. Mesenchyme cells are said to be *pluripotent*, indicating that they may differentiate into a wide variety of cell types, including vessel-, cavity- and duct-lining epithelial cells of mesodermal origin.

The sections opposite

Section A. The forebrain vesicle with its contained cavity, the future third ventricle, is separated from the overlying ectoderm by loose head mesenchyme. The ventrolateral angles of the vesicle have grown out to form primitive eye-cups which have induced the formation of the lens placode in the overlying ectoderm. Mesenchymal condensations, the future oculomotor muscles, are seen near the eye-cup.

Section B. The midbrain vesicle with its contained cavity, the future aqueduct, is surrounded by loose head mesenchyme. The notochord lies ventral to the midbrain, separating it from the flattened endoderm-lined cavity of the primitive pharynx. Laterally, the pharyngeal endoderm is covered with condensed lateral plate mesoderm which extends to the overlying ectoderm. No coelomic cavity is developed in this part of the lateral plate mesoderm, which, reinforced by neural crest material, forms a series of curved bars, the pharyngeal arches, in the ventrolateral walls of the pharynx. Between successive pharyngeal arches, ectodermal depressions and endodermal outpouchings approach each other, forming a series of pharyngeal (branchial) clefts and pouches respectively. The splanchnopleuric ventral wall or floor of the early pharynx also forms the roof of the primitive pericardial cavity which, elsewhere, is bounded by somatopleure.

Section C. The hindbrain vesicle with its contained cavity, the future fourth ventricle, is bounded dorsally by a thinning roof plate. Ventral to the hindbrain lies the notochord, which structures are flanked by mesodermal somites, continuous laterally with the intermediate mesoderm. This relationship of neural tube, notochord, somite and intermediate mesoderm is found at all succeeding trunk levels. The endodermal lining of the foregut is covered with splanchnopleuric mesoderm which continues as dorsal and ventral mesenteries and, thus, separates the two sides of the coelomic cavity at this level. The ventral mesentery is a derivative of the septum transversum which has swung ventral to the foregut during head-fold formation.

Section D. At the level of the primitive umbilicus, a dorsal mesentery suspends the midgut, and from its antimesenteric border the vitellointestinal duct passes through the umbilical cord to become continuous with the definitive yolk sac. The intraembryonic coelom is continuous with a part of the extraembryonic coelom which persists in the embryonic end of the umbilical cord and into which a physiological hernia of the midgut extends in later development.

Section E. The hindgut is suspended by a simple dorsal mesentery. The coelom is continuous ventrally across the midline. Ventrally the allantoic diverticulum is seen in section as it passes towards the caudal margin of the umbilicus.

4-week Embryo

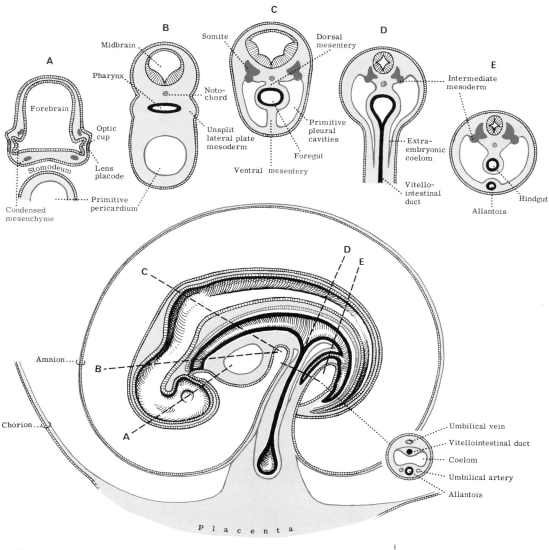

A

Forebrain

Optic cup

Stomodeum

Condensed mesenchyme

Lens placode

B

Midbrain

Pharynx

Noto-chord

Unsplit lateral plate mesoderm

Primitive pericardium

C

Somite

Dorsal mesentery

Primitive pleural cavities

Foregut

Ventral mesentery

D

Extra-embryonic coelom

Vitello-intestinal duct

E

Intermediate mesoderm

Hindgut

Allantois

Amnion

Chorion

Umbilical vein

Vitellointestinal duct

Coelom

Umbilical artery

Allantois

Placenta

4½-week Embryo

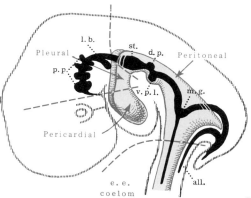

PRIMITIVE COELOMIC REGIONS
(labelled in red)
e.e. - extraembryonic

PRINCIPAL ENDODERMAL REGIONS

p. p. - pharyngeal pouches
l. b. - lung bud
st.   - stomach
d. p. - dorsal pancreas
v. p. l.- ventral pancreas and liver
m. g. - midgut loop
all.   - allantois

Pleural

l. b.

p. p.

st.

d. p.

Peritoneal

v. p. l.

m. g.

Pericardial

e.e. coelom

all.

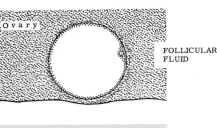

FOLLICULAR
FLUID

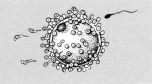

TUBAL
FLUID

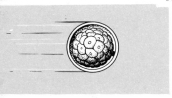

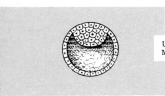

UTERINE
MILK

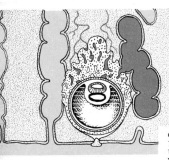

CYTOLYTIC
PRODUCTS,
UTERINE
MILK and
BLOOD

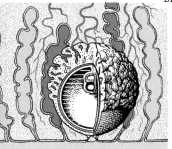

Nutrition

While in the ovarian follicle, the growing oocyte obtains its nutritional requirements from the vessels of the theca interna via the granulosa cell layers and the zona pellucida. Food reserves (yolk) are scanty, and, during fertilization, cleavage and blastocyst formation, nutritional support is obtained by diffusion of tubal secretions and uterine milk, at first through the zona pellucida. Carbon dioxide fixation and pyruvate are essential to early cleavage.

With the elaboration of syncytiotrophoblast, the blastocyst erodes maternal tissues and forms a ragged implantation cavity in the decidua. Within the cavity, the blastocyst is in a fluid medium consisting of extravasated blood, uterine milk and the cytolytic products which follow the breakdown of surface and glandular epithelia, decidual cells and vascular endothelium. The syncytiotrophoblast engulfs this material (*histotroph*).

The early embryo depends upon the passage of nutrients derived from the histotroph through the chorion to the extraembryonic coelom and then to the intraembryonic coelom and through the amnion and yolk sac to their respective cavities; while it is open, the neurenteric canal facilitates exchange between them, the gut and the neural canal. The closure of communications between cavities and the demands of the enlarging embryo make necessary the development of an embryonic circulation (p. 149) and of an extraembryonic system to support it.

As the conceptus enlarges, *histotrophic nutrition* diminishes and *haemotrophic nutrition* begins. This entails the apposition of extraembryonic membranes, and their contained blood vessels, with uterine tissues, so that physiological exchanges between the embryo and the mother may occur (i.e. the formation of a *placenta*). The early human placenta is formed by apposition of the chorion (vascularized by allantoic vessels) with the walls of the implantation cavity. Later it is restricted to the decidua basalis and its apposed chorion.

The walls of the implantation cavity consist of exposed decidual cells, eroded uterine glands and blood vessels. The surrounding stroma shows an increase in vascularity, oedema and decidual reaction. The implantation cavity and eroded glands become filled with extravasated blood.

Although syncytiotrophoblast extends over the whole conceptus, it remains thicker over the embryonic pole, where it is in contact with the richly vascular decidua basalis. The syncytium erodes and replaces the decidua surrounding it. *Lacunae* now appear within the syncytium and coalesce to form an intercommunicating system of spaces separated by irregular syncytial *trabeculae*. Eroding syncytium taps maternal capillaries and venous sinusoids so that blood enters the *labyrinthine space* where, initially, it forms stagnant pools. With expansion of the conceptus, the lacunae enlarge and coalesce to form an *intervillous space* between the larger, radially disposed, syncytial trabeculae. The radial trabeculae are soon invaded by columns of cells from the cytotrophoblast to form *villous stems*. When the tips of the cytotrophoblastic columns reach the outer wall of the intervillous space (*basal plate*), they spread tangentially to meet and fuse with similar expansions from adjacent villous stems and form an incomplete *trophoblastic shell*. *Syncytiotrophoblast* is thus divided into a layer lining the intervillous space and an incomplete layer outside the trophoblastic shell.

Meanwhile, the chorionic ends of the villous stems are invaded by a central core of chorionic somatopleuric mesoderm in which fetal blood vessels develop and make connection with umbilical (allantoic) vessels from the connecting stalk. The mesodermal invasion of the villous stems does not reach the trophoblastic shell. *Cytotrophoblast* is thus found in the inner wall of the intervillous space (*chorionic plate*), as a single layer covering the mesodermal cores of the villous stems, in solid columns at the tips of the villous stems and, finally, in the trophoblastic shell. At this stage the rapidly expanding intervillous space is lined by syncytium, outside which lies cytotrophoblast. Crossing the space radially are the villous stems, which are interconnected by irregular persistent trabeculae. Thus, from the outset, the human placenta is essentially *labyrinthine*.

Numerous finger-like projections of syncytium now extend from the villous stems, and from the chorionic plate between the stems, into the expanding intervillous space. These *true villi* increase in size and are invaded successively by cytotrophoblast and vessel-forming mesoderm. They superimpose a villous character on the pre-existing labyrinth. However, a return towards the labyrinthine form soon follows as syncytial fusion occurs between the tips of neighbouring villi or between villi and the syncytium of the basal plate.

At this stage, therefore, maternal blood percolates through the interstices of a sponge-like framework which surrounds the whole of the chorionic sac but is thicker at the embryonic pole. As gestation advances, the blood supply of the expanding decidua capsularis is reduced. The underlying villous stems and true villi become shorter and sparser, and eventually disappear. This process continues until the stems and villi are confined to a disc-shaped area of chorion covering the embryonic pole and apposed to the decidua basalis. This area, which has the chorionic attachment of the umbilical cord on its embryonic aspect, is called the *chorion frondosum*. With the decidua basalis it forms the definitive placenta. The remainder of the chorionic sac, denuded of stems and villi, presents a smooth surface externally and is called the *chorion laeve*.

The intervillous space of the chorion frondosum soon becomes incompletely divided into 15–20 *cotyledonary bays*. Each bay contains a major villous stem, subsidiary stems and true villi. As adjacent bays expand, with interstitial growth of the overlying trophoblastic shell, tissue persists between them in the form of septa which project from the basal plate towards the chorionic plate. The septa are covered with syncytium and contain prolongations of the trophoblastic shell and decidua basalis.

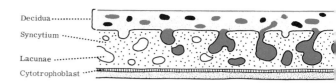

Decidua
Syncytium
Lacunae
Cytotrophoblast

Development is shown from left to right as well as from above downwards

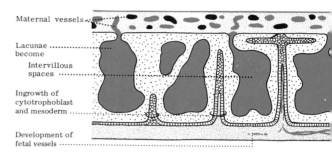

Maternal vessels
Lacunae become Intervillous spaces
Ingrowth of cytotrophoblast and mesoderm
Development of fetal vessels

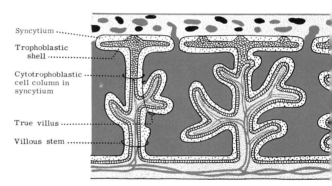

Syncytium
Trophoblastic shell
Cytotrophoblastic cell column in syncytium
True villus
Villous stem

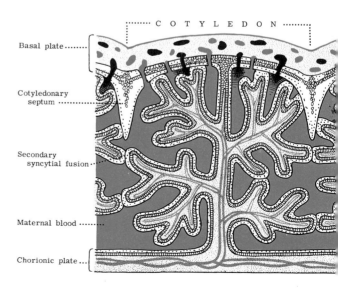

COTYLEDON
Basal plate
Cotyledonary septum
Secondary syncytial fusion
Maternal blood
Chorionic plate

At first the maternal blood in the lacunar system is stagnant, but soon there is an ebb-and-flow movement. As more capillaries and sinusoids are eroded, it develops into a slow percolation through the intervillous space. Progressively larger vessels are eroded but it is not until comparatively late that the large spiral arteries open into the intervillous space through the irregular gaps in the trophoblastic shell. In the mature placenta a number of veins and spiral arteries open into each cotyledon, their orifices being randomly distributed over the basal plate. The arterial orifices are narrow and often partially occluded by endothelial thickening and by cytotrophoblastic cells. Although specific paths for the circulation of maternal blood in the intervillous space have been proposed, the evidence is unconvincing. During its slow passage through the fine spaces of the labyrinth there must be considerable admixture between the blood which enters in discrete spurts and that which leaves for the low-pressure pelvic venous system.

In the early placenta, the fetal and maternal bloodstreams are separated by a placental membrane consisting of fetal endothelium, a thick layer of villous mesoderm, a layer of cytotrophoblast and a fairly thick layer of syncytium. The tissue separating the two bloodstreams is reduced as pregnancy advances. After mid-pregnancy the villous cytotrophoblast largely disappears and the villous syncytium is reduced to a fine covering; the endothelium of the enlarging fetal vessels approaches its inner surface. This increases the efficiency of placental transmission but later in pregnancy is somewhat offset by the degenerative changes (fibrinoid deposition, calcification, endothelial proliferation) which occur in some villi.

As the placenta ages, the trophoblastic shell and the residual syncytium outside it become thinned and form characteristic giant cells. An amorphous fibrinoid material appears at the junction between fetal and maternal tissues, in the chorionic plate and in some villous stems. The placenta achieves its full thickness by mid-pregnancy but continues to increase in circumference until late pregnancy.

At term the placenta is 15–20 cm in diameter, about 3 cm in thickness and 500 g in weight. The fetal aspect is smooth and the umbilical cord is inserted somewhat off centre. From it, the umbilical vessels radiate in the chorionic mesoderm. Overlying this and continued over the umbilical cord is the amnion. The amnion may be fused with the placental chorionic mesoderm and, beyond the margin of the placenta, is fused with the mesoderm of the chorion laeve. A small persistent yolk sac is sometimes found between the amnion and the chorion near the placental end of the umbilical cord.

Separation of the placenta occurs through the attenuated decidua basalis and, after delivery, the irregular maternal surface shows 15–20 convex cotyledons separated by grooves. The exposed surface is made up of basal plate, and the grooves overlie the bases of the cotyledonary septa.

The placenta is an organ for physiological exchanges between fetus and mother. It also functions as a complex endocrine gland and as a store for certain metabolites. The physiological exchanges involve the passage of nutrients, oxygen, water, hormones and antibodies from mother to fetus, and carbon dioxide, water, nitrogenous waste products and hormones from fetus to mother.

In general, gases and some substances of low molecular weight in solution pass by simple diffusion, glucose and fatty acids by facilitated diffusion, electrolytes, amino acids and water-soluble vitamins by active transport and macromolecules by selective pinocytosis. Selective pinocytosis, for example, permits the passage of maternal immunoglobulins which confer passive immunity on the fetus, while denying that of some potentially deleterious macromolecules of the same or smaller size. Some glucose is taken up by the placenta and converted into glycogen and fat which are stored; similarly, some fatty acids are incorporated into neutral fat in the placenta.

There is little or no transfer of complex sugars, of proteins including protein hormones, or of lipids, phospholipids or lipoproteins. Transport of protein-bound or conjugated steroid hormones is very slow but that of free steroids is rapid. There are in fact few substances that are unable to pass the placenta in detectable amounts and *caution is thus necessary in prescribing for pregnant women.*

Leakage also occurs, so fetal red blood cells and fragments of trophoblast are found in the maternal circulation. In this way the *Rhesus antigen* is transmitted from a Rhesus-positive fetus to a Rhesus-negative mother. When it occurs, the mother is sensitized and produces antibodies which cross the barrier, destroy fetal blood cells and cause haemolytic disease of the newborn.

The placenta also provides an impassable barrier for the majority of micro-organisms which may be present in the mother's blood. There are, however, important exceptions; e.g. maternal *rubella* in the first 3 months of pregnancy may affect the fetus and cause congenital anomalies of the eye and heart. In maternal *syphilis*, the spirochaete may cross the placental barrier in the second half of pregnancy and cause congenital syphilis.

As an endocrine gland the cytotrophoblast produces a gonadotrophin-releasing hormone (GnRH) whilst the syncytiotrophoblast produces human chorionic gonadotrophin (hCG), oestrogens, progesterone, β-endorphins and human chorionic somatomammotropin (hCS). Formerly known as placental lactogen, the protein hCS has both prolactin- and growth-hormone-like actions: it may stimulate the production of prolactin-inhibiting factor by the hypothalamus so that lactation is inhibited during pregnancy.

The Placenta at term

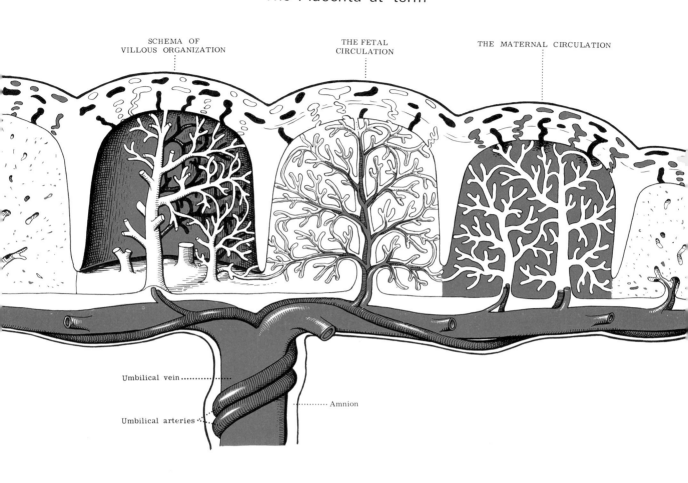

SCHEMA OF VILLOUS ORGANIZATION

THE FETAL CIRCULATION

THE MATERNAL CIRCULATION

Umbilical vein

Umbilical arteries

Amnion

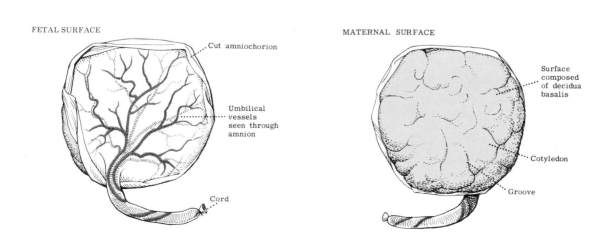

FETAL SURFACE

Cut amniochorion

Umbilical vessels seen through amnion

Cord

MATERNAL SURFACE

Surface composed of decidua basalis

Cotyledon

Groove

By stimulating the corpus luteum to produce oestrogens and progesterone, hCG maintains the pregnancy until the secretion of those hormones by the placenta can assume the role. This controlled changeover normally occurs at about the time of the third suppressed menstrual period (a common time for abortion); little hCG is produced thereafter. Rising hCG levels in early pregnancy permit its detection in maternal urine by biological or immunological methods. After the third month, during which blood levels of ovarian progesterone have fallen, those of placental oestrogens and progesterone both rise steadily for at least 5 months. During the last month the actions of oestrogens dominate the picture: they increase the sensitivity of the myometrium to oxytocin and prostaglandins, hormones which play some part in the initiation of labour.

Placentae may be classified according to general shape, fine structure, intimacy of fusion between extraembryonic membranes and maternal tissues, source of fetal blood vessels and whether maternal tissue is shed with the placenta and membranes. In these terms the human placenta would be described as *discoidal*, *labyrinthine* (and *secondarily villous*), *haemochorial*, *chorioallantoic* and *deciduate*.

Uterine placental sites

The placenta may be formed at any point on the walls of the uterine cavity. The commonest site is on the posterior wall, then, in descending order of frequency, on the anterior wall, the sides, near the internal os and finally at the fundus. Of these, only sites near the internal os are of clinical significance, and then the term *placenta praevia* is used. The internal os may be partially or completely covered—lateral or central placenta praevia. When dilatation of the cervix occurs in labour a placenta praevia will partially detach, exposing torn maternal vessels and causing antepartum haemorrhage.

Twins and their placentae

Fraternal (non-identical) twins normally have separate membrane systems and placentae but secondary fusion between the chorionic sacs may occur. Identical twins show a variable membrane relationship. Separation of early blastomeres results in separate membranes and placentae as in fraternal twins. Division of the inner cell mass gives a single common chorion and placental mass, within which there may be two separate amniotic sacs or, occasionally, a single common sac.

Abnormal placentae

Normally the chorionic part of the human placenta is developed from the disc-shaped chorion frondosum, but variations in the distribution of the chorion frondosum may occur, resulting in bizarre forms. Persistence over most of the chorionic sac results in a *placenta diffusa* (normal in the pig). Persistence of an equatorial band results in a *zonary placenta* (normal in the dog and the cat). Other variations include the *bidiscoidal placenta*, the subdivisions of which receive separate terminal branches of the umbilical cord (normal in the monkey), and the *placenta succenturiata* in which one or more cotyledons are separate from the main placenta. The succenturiate lobe is supplied by vessels crossing the chorion from the main placental mass. Such vessels may be damaged when the membranes rupture early in labour, causing fetal haemorrhage. In addition, a succenturiate lobe may be retained within the uterus after delivery of the main placenta and membranes. Such a retained lobe may interfere with the immediate closure of maternal vessels, causing postpartum haemorrhage or may be a focus for subsequent infection of the birth canal.

Occasionally, excessive invasion of the uterine wall by the trophoblast results in penetration of the decidua basalis and invasion of the myometrium to form an abnormally adherent *placenta accreta*. The growth of the trophoblast may also be excessive, with loss of the embryo and the formation of a polycystic mass (*hydatidiform mole*). This or, rarely, an otherwise normal placenta may undergo malignant change (*chorionepithelioma*).

Abnormalities of the umbilical cord

The vessels of the umbilical cord are considerably longer than its covering and take a spiral and looped course. The mucoidal connective tissue is thicker over the loops, resulting in surface irregularities termed 'false knots'. True knots also occur but are uncommon, and rarely tighten sufficiently to interfere with fetal circulation.

The umbilical cord may be abnormally short. It is usually inserted somewhat eccentrically into the fetal surface of the placenta. Variations include a *marginal insertion* (*battledore placenta*) and a *velamentous insertion*. In the latter the umbilical vessels arborize in the chorion before entering the placental margin and may be damaged in labour.

Extrauterine pregnancy

Tissues other than the endometrium may receive and support the blastocyst in an extrauterine (*ectopic*) pregnancy. The commonest site is the uterine tube. The trophoblast burrows into the wall of the tube, which undergoes a miniature decidual reaction. The lumen of the tube is obliterated and its thin wall stretched by the expanding conceptus. This frequently leads to rupture of the tube and tubal vessels, with intraperitoneal haemorrhage. Rupture occurs early in isthmic, and later in cornual or ampullary pregnancies. Alternatively, the conceptus may detach and die, being either extruded into the peritoneal or uterine cavities, or retained within the uterine tube. On rare occasions slow rupture or thinning of the ampullary end of the tube may result in secondary implantation in the peritoneal cavity.

TWIN MEMBRANES

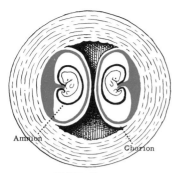

Amnion   Chorion

FRATERNAL TWINS

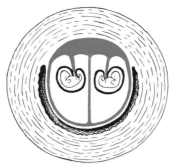

IDENTICAL TWINS

single amnion

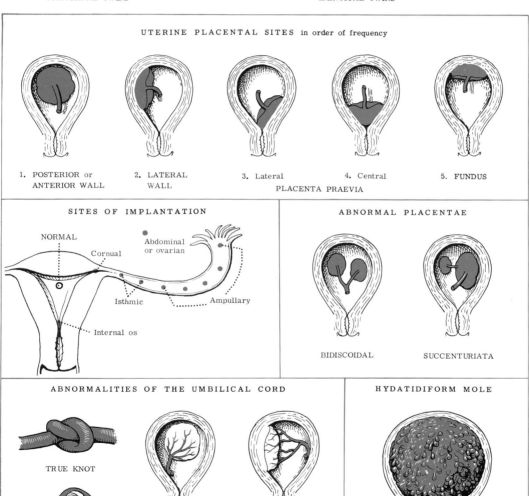

UTERINE PLACENTAL SITES in order of frequency

1. POSTERIOR or ANTERIOR WALL

2. LATERAL WALL

3. Lateral

4. Central

PLACENTA PRAEVIA

5. FUNDUS

SITES OF IMPLANTATION

NORMAL

Cornual

Abdominal or ovarian

Isthmic

Ampullary

Internal os

ABNORMAL PLACENTAE

BIDISCOIDAL

SUCCENTURIATA

ABNORMALITIES OF THE UMBILICAL CORD

TRUE KNOT

FALSE KNOT

BATTLEDORE PLACENTA

VELAMENTOUS INSERTION

HYDATIDIFORM MOLE

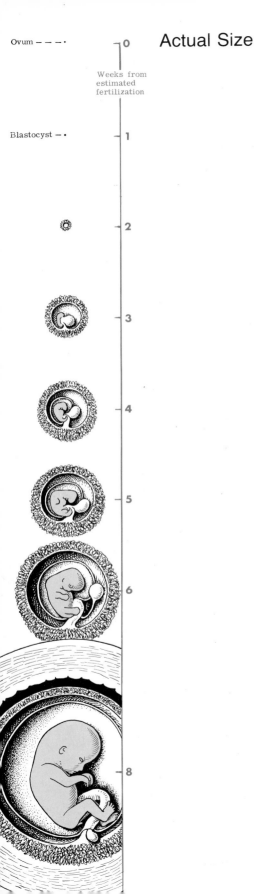

Ovum – – –·

Weeks from
estimated
fertilization

Blastocyst – ·

0

1

2

3

4

5

6

8

Actual Size

Developmental Levels

It is usual in obstetric practice to count the human gestation period from the first day of the last menstrual period (LMP). The age of a fetus estimated in this way (*menstrual age*) is usually some 14 days more than its *ovulation age*. The *coital age* approximates (2–3 days) to the ovulation age. *Fertilization age* would be ideal but this cannot be determined precisely in vivo and may be as much as 4 days less than coital age.

Life in utero consists of three phases—pre-embryonic (the first 2½ weeks), embryonic (until the end of week 8) and fetal (from 8 weeks until term).

The *pre-embryonic phase* includes cleavage, blastocyst formation, and the formation of the extraembryonic membranes and the presomite embryo. After fertilization, the first 3–4 days are occupied with transport down the uterine tube and cleavage to form a morula. By 7–8 days, implantation of the early blastocyst has begun. By 14 days, the early presomite embryo is a circular bilaminar disc with prechordal plate, primitive streak, primitive node, notochordal process and cloacal membrane. At 18 days the embryo is about to enter the somite stage. It is a trilaminar, pear-shaped disc with a neural plate, a neural groove and early head and tail folds.

The *embryonic phase* begins with the somite stage, which occupies the next 10 days. During this stage, head-, tail- and lateral-fold formation occur and the mesodermal somites are laid down, the number present being used as an index of development.

By the 7-somite stage, closure of the neural tube has begun and the cephalic enlargement of the neural plate is marked. At the 10-somite stage the three primary cerebral dilatations are obvious. Closure of the neural tube has progressed caudally beyond the region of formed somites and cranially to the midbrain region. The tube remains unclosed at the anterior and posterior neuropores. The oral membrane forms the floor of the stomodeum, which is bounded cranially by the anterior projecting edge of the neural plate (later the bulge of the forebrain) and caudally by the bulge of the pericardium. Laterally the stomodeum is bounded on each side by a swelling which has appeared in the angle between the neural plate and the pericardium. This is the *mandibular prominence* of the *first pharyngeal arch*. As successive arches appear, the pericardium is progressively removed from the caudal margin of the stomodeum.

By the 14-somite stage, the neuropores are much reduced in size and folding has progressed so that a wide, elliptical, primitive umbilicus may be distinguished. Caudal to the first pharyngeal arch, which bounds the stomodeum (S) is a wide, *first pharyngeal groove*. Caudal again is the prominent *second (hyoid) arch* and the narrower *second groove*. An ectodermal thickening is present dorsal to the second groove. This is the *otic placode* and is the precursor of the membranous labyrinth. Soon it is to sink into the floor of a depression—the *otic pit*—which pinches off from the surface and forms the *otic vesicle*.

Towards the end of the somite stage the neuropores close, and folding is completed with the formation of a well-defined umbilicus, umbilical cord and tail. The embryo has the typical comma-shaped form with a marked primary embryonic curve. Succeeding pharyngeal arches appear and the otic vesicle sinks into head mesenchyme so that it is no longer seen through the ectoderm. An evagination of the forebrain—the *optic vesicle*—makes its appearance beneath the head ectoderm. It is the precursor of the retina and epithelia of the iris and ciliary body.

With the passing of the somite stage, changes of external form occur more slowly, and the establishment of embryonic age is facilitated by an accurate menstrual or coital history. Often this is not available and then an approximation has to be made from a consideration of certain standard measurements and the general topography of the embryo. The former include crown–heel (CH; standing) length, crown–rump (CR; sitting) length and neck–rump length. The last-named is used when the embryo has an unusually acute cervical flexure. As a guide, the embryo is 5 mm CR at the end of the somite stage, and 8 mm at 5 weeks. It increases 1 mm per day until 8 weeks and 1.5 mm per day thereafter. As a broad guide for the fetus of 3–4 months:

$$(\text{age in months})^2 = \text{CR length in cm}$$

and thereafter:

$$\text{age in months} \times 5 = \text{CH length in cm}$$

During the second month the primary embryonic curve is gradually modified by the growth of the nervous system, with the development of the cervical, pontine and midbrain flexures and the expansion of the forebrain. The surface elevations caused by the underlying somites become less prominent and, finally, disappear. *Forelimb buds* appear dorsal to the pericardium and, somewhat later, *hindlimb buds* appear, dorsal to the posterior line of attachment of the umbilical cord. Throughout its development the forelimb bud is in advance of the hindlimb bud, each beginning as a conical projection somewhat flattened dorsoventrally. Constrictions demarcating the three main limb segments soon appear, followed by the early digits, which have the form of divergent rays united by thick webs. By 2 months the digits have separated and the preaxial digits are prominent.

The hyoid arch remains prominent but subsequent arches become flattened or overgrown by tissue from the edges of the hyoid arch and pericardium, forming a smooth contour for the neck. The margins of the first ectodermal groove develop a series of elevations which fuse to form the external ear.

With further expansion of the brain and head, modification of the cervical curvature, retrogression of the tail and development of the face and eyes, the embryo assumes a characteristically human form by 2 months.

The *fetal* and *postnatal phases* (p. 162) are characterized by growth and changes in proportion rather than by the appearance of new features.

External Form

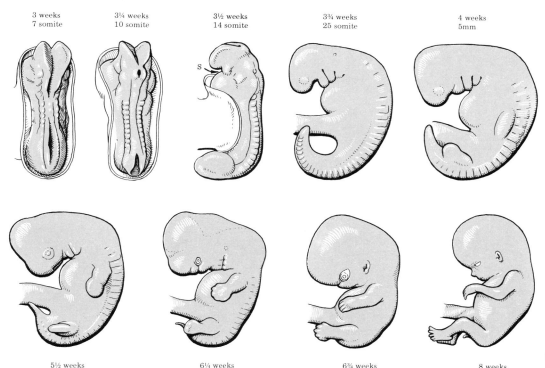

3 weeks	3¼ weeks	3½ weeks	3¾ weeks	4 weeks
7 somite	10 somite	14 somite	25 somite	5mm

5½ weeks	6¼ weeks	6¾ weeks	8 weeks
10mm	13½mm	17mm	30mm

The Pharynx, Face, Respiratory System and Endocrine Glands

In all chordates the development of the face and pharynx centres upon the *pharyngeal arches*, a series of thickenings which appear in the side wall of the foregut and grow ventrally. On the inside, *pharyngeal pouches* grow out between arches and are lined with *endoderm*. On the outside, surface *ectoderm* dips into *pharyngeal grooves*. The endodermal pouches and ectodermal grooves approach each other between arches and form *closing membranes*. In fishes the arches develop vascular gills and the membranes break down to form gill clefts so that water, which has entered via the mouth, can leave the pharynx via the clefts and oxygenate blood in the gills. In terrestrial animals, including man, the membranes do not normally rupture, and grooves and pouches have lost this role. The pharynx, however, remains concerned with oxygenation and respiratory exchange because the lungs develop from its floor. It is also important because of the glands which form from pharyngeal endoderm in all vertebrates.

In man, tissue over the forebrain becomes the *frontonasal prominence* which will form the brow and the nose. The nostrils will develop in it as bilateral ectodermal thickenings—the *nasal placodes* (which will form the smell epithelium)—sink into pits. In all, six pharyngeal arches appear in succession but the fifth is transitory or absent. The first pharyngeal arch to appear is called *mandibular* because the mandible will develop in it. When it meets its fellow of the opposite side and forms the lower jaw, the oral membrane breaks down so that surface ectoderm and gut endoderm meet in the oral cavity. In addition to forming one side of the lower jaw, each first arch has a *maxillary prominence* which grows across to fuse with its fellow and with the frontonasal prominence to form the upper jaw. Palatal processes from the maxillary prominences meet to fuse in the midline and separate the nasal and oral cavities. The eye develops in relation to the forebrain between the frontonasal and maxillary prominences. The external ear forms around the dorsal end of the first groove. The rest of that groove and all succeeding grooves fill out to give a smooth contour to the face and neck.

The connective tissue core of each arch contains a bar of *cartilage*. The bar in the first arch forms ear ossicles and the basis for the mandible. The second bar forms ear ossicles and the upper part of the hyoid bone at the base of the tongue. Succeeding bars form the rest of the hyoid bone and the laryngeal cartilages.

The first pharyngeal pouch mainly forms a diverticulum which expands into the auditory (*Eustachian*) tube and grows around the ear ossicles as the middle ear cavity. The closing membrane between the first two arches thus becomes the ear drum. The endoderm of the remaining pouches forms the epithelia (*parenchyma*) of the tonsil, thymus and parathyroid glands. The *stroma* (Gk = bedding) of glands is derived from surrounding connective tissue.

The pharyngeal pouches do not reach the midline ventrally. Here a number of structures form from the arches. The endodermal covering and connective tissues of the anterior two-thirds of the tongue form from the first arch and those of the posterior one-third from the third arch. Between them an endodermal diverticulum grows down into the connective tissue of the midline of the neck and forms the epithelium of the thyroid gland. Behind the tongue another midline endodermal diverticulum grows down from the pharynx between the rest of the foregut and the heart. Two lung buds appear at its lower end and the larynx forms around its upper end. The pharynx thus retains roles in both the development of glands and in respiration.

The pituitary gland, too, is related to the pharynx, or, more precisely, to the oral membrane. However, its parenchyma derives from ectoderm rather than from endoderm. The ectoderm is derived from two sources—the anterior pituitary (*adenohypophysis*) forming from a recess near the oral membrane called Rathke's pouch, and the posterior pituitary (*neurohypophysis*) forming from a related recess in the floor of the forebrain. Again, the stroma is derived from surrounding connective tissue.

The other major endocrine glands form in the abdomen.

Development of Face and Neck

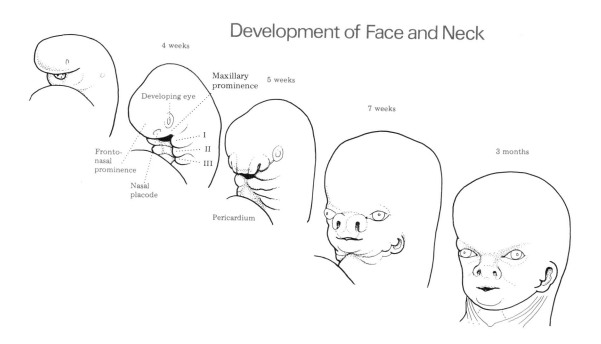

4 weeks

Developing eye

Maxillary prominence

5 weeks

7 weeks

3 months

Fronto-nasal prominence

I
II
III

Nasal placode

Pericardium

Pharynx

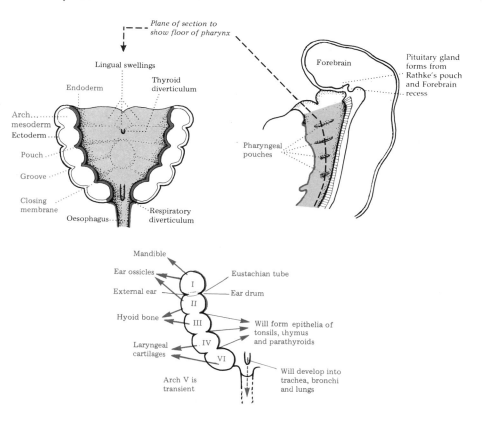

Plane of section to show floor of pharynx

Lingual swellings

Endoderm

Thyroid diverticulum

Arch mesoderm
Ectoderm

Pouch

Groove

Closing membrane

Oesophagus

Respiratory diverticulum

Forebrain

Pituitary gland forms from Rathke's pouch and Forebrain recess

Pharyngeal pouches

Mandible

Ear ossicles

External ear

Eustachian tube

Ear drum

I

II

Hyoid bone

III

Will form epithelia of tonsils, thymus and parathyroids

Laryngeal cartilages

IV

VI

Arch V is transient

Will develop into trachea, bronchi and lungs

67

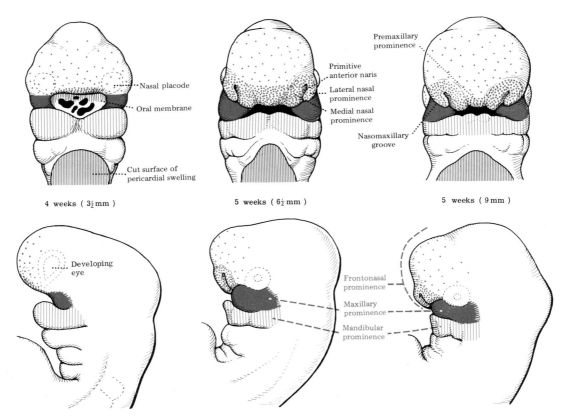

4 weeks (3½ mm)   5 weeks (6½ mm)   5 weeks (9 mm)

Nasal placode

Oral membrane

Cut surface of
pericardial swelling

Premaxillary
prominence

Primitive
anterior naris

Lateral nasal
prominence

Medial nasal
prominence

Nasomaxillary
groove

Developing
eye

Frontonasal
prominence

Maxillary
prominence

Mandibular
prominence

The face

In an early somite embryo the intact *oral membrane* is bound cranially by the anterior edge of the neural plate and neural ridge, caudally by the pericardial swelling and laterally by the *mandibular prominence* of each first pharyngeal arch. With the closure of the anterior neuropore, the neural plate forms the bulging forebrain. Most of the neural ridge, which surrounded the neural plate, is then found in the angle between the neural tube and surface ectoderm as neural crest (p. 125). However, the part adjacent to the oral membrane remains adherent to the floor of the forebrain and forms the roof of the *stomodeum*. By the late somite stage, the oral membrane has broken down, establishing continuity between the stomodeum and the primitive pharynx, and another swelling—the *maxillary prominence*—has extended towards the stomodeum from the dorsal end of each first arch. The stomodeum is now bounded cranially by the frontal bulge of the forebrain, laterally by the maxillary prominences and caudally by the mandibular prominences which extend towards each other and merge in the midline to form the primitive lower jaw and lip.

Bilateral ectodermal thickenings—the *nasal placodes*—appear above the lateral angles of the stomo-deum. Accumulation of mesenchyme around each placode causes the elevation of a horseshoe-shaped area of surrounding ectoderm. The limbs of the horseshoe are termed the *medial* and the *lateral nasal prominences*. The nasal prominences, together with an intervening *premaxillary prominence* and the bulge of the forebrain, constitute the *frontonasal prominence*. The nasal placode at this stage forms the floor of an *olfactory pit* which is incompletely surrounded by the nasal prominences.

The mandibular, maxillary and frontonasal prominences are each elevations of ectoderm overlying an accumulation of condensed mesenchyme. Adjacent prominences are separated by superficial ectodermal grooves, their 'fusion' usually entailing a filling out of the intervening groove as they become continuous, with some admixture of their mesenchymatous cores. In some sites, however, this process is preceded by true epithelial fusion, with the result that epithelial cells become buried in mesenchyme along the line of fusion.

The lateral nasal prominence separates the deepening olfactory pit from the site of the developing eye, being itself separated from the triangular maxillary prominence by an ectodermal *nasomaxillary groove*. As fusion proceeds between the maxillary prominence and the lateral nasal prominence, a solid rod of epithelial cells sinks into the subjacent mesenchyme.

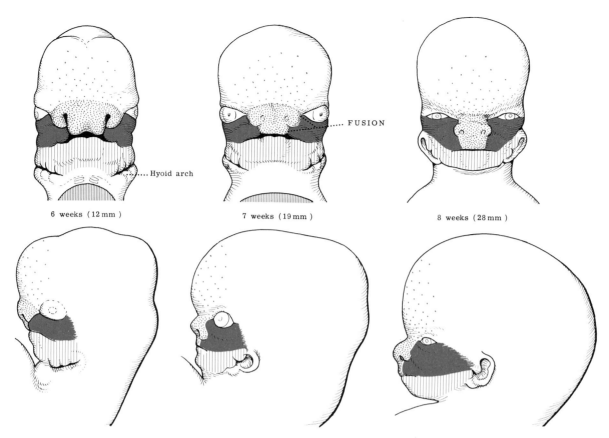

6 weeks (12 mm)   7 weeks (19 mm) ..... FUSION   8 weeks (28 mm)

..... Hyoid arch

The ends of the rod grow, establishing secondary connections with the developing conjunctival sac and with the lateral wall of the deepening olfactory pit (*nasal sac*). Subsequently, canalization of the rod establishes the *nasolacrimal sac* and *duct*. The apex of each maxillary prominence continues to grow medially, and crosses the end of the lateral nasal prominence to reach the medial nasal and premaxillary prominences. For a while a groove persists between the advancing elevation of the maxillary prominence and the premaxillary prominence. Slowly this groove is filled out and their mesenchymatous cores become continuous, i.e. they 'fuse'. Thus, a continuous upper lip is established. It is often considered that the lateral parts of the upper lip are derived from the maxillary prominence and that a median strip is derived from the premaxillary prominence. However, some hold that the maxillary prominences continue to grow medially until they meet, fusing in the midline and excluding the premaxillary prominence from the surface. The wide primitive oral fissure is reduced by progressive fusion between the maxillary and mandibular prominences with the formation of the cheeks. The lips and cheeks are invaded by second pharyngeal arch mesenchyme which forms the facial muscles.

The further development of the face mainly entails changes in proportion and relative position. The forebrain continues to expand, and the eyes, initially directed laterally, gradually become directed anteriorly. The nasal sacs are at first widely separated but come closer together as the intervening tissue—the *primitive nasal septum*—thins and the medial nasal prominences fuse. At the same time a transverse groove appears, defining the upper limit of the external nose and separating it from the frontal area. The *anterior nares* become plugged with proliferated epithelium. The *external ear*, which develops around the margins of the first ectodermal groove, is at first caudal to the developing face but it gradually approaches and passes above the level of the mouth.

The sites of emergence of nerves from the developing central nervous system are determined by the inductive influence of surrounding masses of mesenchyme. Thus, in general, the derivatives of the *frontonasal prominence* are supplied by the ophthalmic nerve, those of the *maxillary prominence* by the maxillary nerve, and those of the *mandibular prominence* by the mandibular nerve. There is, however, no rigid demarcation of separate zones, overlapping of territories occurring where 'fusion' of processes has occurred. With the relatively enormous expansion of the human forebrain, cutaneous branches of the cervical nerves also encroach upon the head.

The nose, palate and hypophysis

The *nasal sacs* are a pair of blind-ended pouches bounded by the medial and lateral nasal prominences. Each sac has a ventral fold from which an epithelial *nasal fin* extends down to the roof of the stomodeum. The maxillary and frontonasal prominences fuse in front of the nasal fins to complete the *anterior nares* and form the *primitive palate* separating the nasal and stomodeal cavities. Above the primitive palate the diverging nasal sacs are separated by a thick *primitive nasal septum*. Behind the primitive palate each nasal fin progressively breaks down until only an *oronasal membrane* separates the nasal sac from the stomodeum. When the oronasal membranes break down, the *posterior nares* or *choanae* are established. At this stage, each posterior naris is bounded by the edge of the primitive nasal septum, the edge of the primitive palate, the maxillary prominence and the roof of the stomodeum.

As a result of differential growth, the roof of the stomodeum becomes progressively more highly arched. The *tongue*, which is developing from the floor of the pharynx, comes into contact with the roof. The maxillary prominences develop medially directed shelf-like outgrowths—the *palatal processes*. Their bases are in the same horizontal plane as the primitive palate but, with continued growth, their advancing edges impinge on the sides of the developing tongue and are deflected downwards. The posterior nares gradually migrate as the *definitive nasal septum* grows downwards and backwards from the angle between the roof of the stomodeum and the back of the premaxillary prominence. Growth is mainly due to proliferation of the midline mesenchyme which separates the epithelial roof of the stomodeum from the forebrain. Mesenchyme from the maxillary prominences, which migrates towards the midline above the epithelial roof of the stomodeum, may contribute to this *septal mesenchyme*. The effect of downward growth of the septum is enhanced by the upward expansion of the nasal fossae on either side of it. Initially, the septum is thick and its expanded lower end is in contact with the dorsum of the tongue. Later it becomes thinner and its mesenchyme condenses. Later still, cartilage and membrane bone make their appearance.

With growth of the neck and the mandibular region, the tongue sinks below the level of the primitive palate so that the palatal processes become free to swing into the horizontal plane. As they continue to grow, the palatal processes fuse with the back of the primitive palate and then with each other, from before backwards, to form the *definitive palate*. At the same time, the lower free edge of the nasal septum grows down to meet the upper surface of the fusing palatal processes and fuses with them, completing the boundaries of the nasal fossae and the oral cavity.

Later, ossification in the mesenchyme of the primitive palate region and of the palatal processes forms the palatine process of the maxilla and the horizontal plate of the palatine bone. Whether or not there are separate premaxillary centres is disputed. The maxillary mesenchyme of the part of the palate behind the posterior edge of the nasal septum and beyond the ossifying zone mainly forms the connective tissue framework of the soft palate and uvula. It is invaded by mesenchyme from other pharyngeal arches which differentiates into palatal musculature. The site of the junction between the palatal processes of maxillary mesenchyme and the primitive palate may be indicated in the adult by the incisive fossa.

The narrow roof and immediately adjacent walls of the nasal fossae are covered by *nasal placode* tissue. This differentiates into *olfactory epithelium* and sends olfactory nerve fibres to the overlying forebrain which develops *olfactory bulbs*. A number of elevations develop on the lateral wall of each nasal fossa and soon coalesce to form the three *nasal conchae*. Towards term and in postnatal life a series of outpouchings appear between the conchae. These invade some of the bones of the nasal skeleton to form the *paranasal sinuses*.

In the head most of the neural ridge becomes neural crest which forms cranial ganglia and migrates into the various prominences as mesenchyme. The neural ridge adjacent to the oral membrane, however, remains adherent to the floor of the forebrain and forms the roof of the stomodeum. As mesenchyme accumulates around this adhering region it becomes isolated in recesses from the stomodeum—*Rathke's pouch* (the *hypophyseal sac*)—and from the forebrain cavity—the *infundibular sac*. After separating from the stomodeum, with differential growth, cytodifferentiation and invasion by mesenchyme to form the stroma, Rathke's pouch forms the *adenohypophysis*. A constant remnant in the roof of the stomodeum forms the *pharyngeal hypophysis*. The infundibular sac closes but remains attached to the *diencephalon* by a stalk and forms the *neurohypophysis*.

Nose and Palate

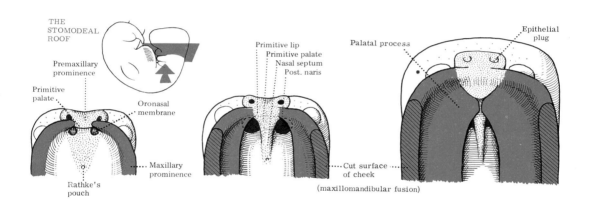

CORONAL SECTIONS

Primitive nasal fossa

Primitive nasal fossa

Olfactory nerve fibres

Eye

Maxillary prominence

Mandibular prominence

Stomodeal cavity

Nasal fin

Olfactory bulb

Forebrain

Nasal septum

Fusion

Palatal process

Tongue

Subsequent fusion

THE STOMODEAL ROOF

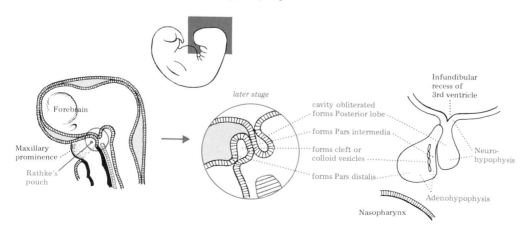

Premaxillary prominence

Primitive palate

Oronasal membrane

Maxillary prominence

Rathke's pouch

Primitive lip
Primitive palate
Nasal septum
Post. naris

Cut surface of cheek

(maxillomandibular fusion)

Palatal process

Epithelial plug

Hypophysis Cerebri

Forebrain

Maxillary prominence

Rathke's pouch

later stage

cavity obliterated forms Posterior lobe

forms Pars intermedia

forms cleft or colloid vesicles

forms Pars distalis

Infundibular recess of 3rd ventricle

Neuro-hypophysis

Adenohypophysis

Nasopharynx

The pharyngeal arches

Under the influence of pharyngeal endoderm and with the inflow of mesenchyme from the cranial part of the neural crest, the unsplit lateral plate mesoderm of the pharyngeal wall forms six curved cylindrical thickenings—*pharyngeal (branchial) arches*—on each side. The arches grow from a region lateral to the hindbrain, through the lateral wall of the pharynx and into the ventral wall where they grow towards their fellows of the opposite side. As the ventral ends of the arches approach the midline they progressively separate the pericardium from the stomodeum. The anterior arches are the first to develop and they remain larger than the others. The first (mandibular) arch, which is also influenced by stomodeal ectoderm, has an additional prominence. The mandibular prominence is at its ventral end and the maxillary prominence develops as an extension from its dorsal end. A general comparison may be made between the human pharyngeal arches and the pharyngeal structures of a jawed fish or generalized vertebrate. The mandibular arch corresponds to the jaws, the second (hyoid) arch to the atypical arch between the spiracle and the first gill cleft, and the remaining arches to the typical gill-bearing (i.e. branchial) arches.

The arches are also represented on the inside of the pharynx. The mandibular prominences of the first arch meet and fuse across the midline. The hyoid arches also meet and fuse. The ventral ends of the succeeding arches fail to reach the midline and are separated by a median swelling of the pharyngeal floor—the *copula*. In the human embryo the fifth arch is only transiently present and its derivatives are not precisely known.

Each arch consists of a mesenchymal core covered externally by ectoderm and internally by endoderm. Contiguous arches are separated externally by *pharyngeal (branchial) grooves* lined with ectoderm and internally by *pharyngeal pouches* lined with endoderm. Between the arches the epithelial linings of the grooves and pouches approach each other and form *closing membranes*. In lower vertebrates the membranes rupture and complete gill clefts are formed. In terrestrial vertebrates, including man, this does not normally occur and the grooves and pouches remain discrete.

In all vertebrates, development of the pharyngeal arches follows the same basic plan. The crest mesenchyme forms connective tissues including, by condensation and then chondrification, a cylindrical *arch cartilage*. The lateral plate mesoderm differentiates into muscle and endothelium. Unlike most muscle related to the gut wall, this muscle is striated. It is therefore designated *special visceral (branchial) muscle*. An *aortic arch artery* develops caudal to the arch cartilage and connects the ventral aorta (aortic sac in the human embryo) with the dorsal aorta of its side. In aquatic vertebrates the aortic arch arteries are the blood vessels which supply the gills. In terrestrial vertebrates, with the advent of lung-breathing, the pattern of aortic arches is subsequently modified as they form the large arteries of the neck and thorax. These modifications entail cell death which is a feature of pharyngeal arch development. A mixed, motor and sensory, *nerve* grows into each arch from the lateral aspect of the hindbrain. The *motor component* innervates the striated pharyngeal arch musculature and is thus classified as a *special visceral efferent (branchiomotor)* component. In primitive vertebrates the *sensory component* branches dorsal to the gill clefts and its divisions supply the caudal and cranial surfaces of the preceding gill cleft (*trema*). The *post-trematic branch* runs with the motor component and supplies the epithelium on the cranial surface of its own arch. The *pretrematic branch* arches over the preceding cleft to reach and supply the epithelium on the caudal surface of the preceding arch. Each arch thus contains its own nerve (motor + post-trematic) and a branch of the nerve of the succeeding arch.

In the human embryo the first arch nerve is the mandibular division of the trigeminal nerve; the second arch nerve is the facial nerve; the third arch nerve is the glossopharyngeal nerve; the fourth arch nerve is the superior laryngeal branch of the vagus nerve; the sixth arch nerve is the recurrent laryngeal branch of the vagus nerve. In man, the arch nerves have branches which pass into the territory of preceding arches. The facial nerve (arch 2) has a greater petrosal branch which supplies the palate (arch 1); the glossopharyngeal nerve (arch 3) has a tympanic branch which supplies the walls of the auditory tube and tympanic cavity (arches 1, 2 and 3); the vagus nerve (arches 4 and 6) has an auricular branch which supplies parts of the pinna, external acoustic meatus and tympanic membrane (arches 1 and 2). However, the relationships and distribution of these branches and of the chorda tympani branch of the facial nerve which supplies the anterior two-thirds of the tongue (arch 1) are not typical of pretrematic nerves and it is doubtful whether they should be considered as homologues.

Ectodermal derivatives

The ectoderm of the first arch forms the epidermis and epidermal derivatives of the lower face and lips, the epithelium of the oral vestibule and gums, the epithelial component of various oral glands, and the enamel organs of the teeth. Certain ectodermal thickenings—*epibranchial placodes*—arise near the dorsal ends of the ectodermal grooves. These placodes sink below the surface, become vesicular and associate with the developing pharyngeal arch nerves. In lower vertebrates these placodes contribute neurons to the sensory ganglia of pharyngeal nerves V, VII, IX and X: they are presumed to contribute neurons concerned with visceral sensation, including taste, to these ganglia in man. The pinna arises by the coalescence of tubercles around the orifice of the first pharyngeal groove. The tragus is derived from the mandibular arch, and the remainder of the pinna from the hyoid arch. The first groove ectoderm contributes to the lining of the external acoustic meatus and the outer epithelium of the tympanic membrane. Development of the first two arches outstrips that of succeeding arches which form the floor of a depression—the *cervical sinus*. Within the sinus the epibranchial placodes sink below the surface, and the third arch overlaps and eventually buries the fourth arch. In subsequent development the first ectodermal groove ventral to the external acoustic meatus is filled out to give a smooth contour to the face. The second groove is represented by the flexure line of the neck. The cervical sinus becomes raised to give a smooth contour to the neck, after which third arch ectoderm is represented over the carotid triangle.

The *parotid gland* develops from a bud which arises near the angle of the wide primitive oral fissure and grows back towards the ear. The bud branches, canalizes and differentiates into glandular tissue. As the cheek forms, a groove on its inner aspect closes over to form the parotid duct. As in other glands, the connective tissue and vessels develop from surrounding mesenchyme.

The submandibular and sublingual glands form similarly but their epithelia are derived from endoderm. A groove running forwards from the origin of the submandibular bud closes over to form the submandibular duct. The sublingual gland arises from a series of buds, most of which retain their own connection with the floor of the mouth.

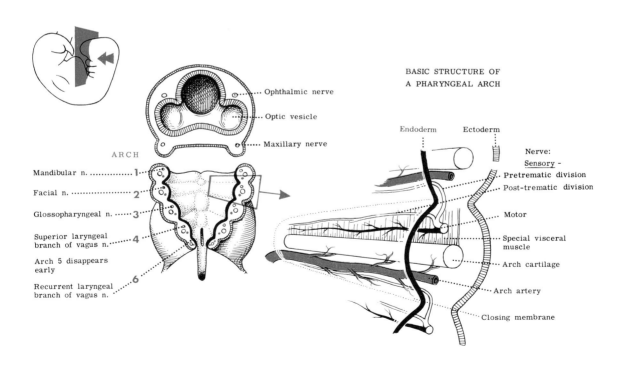

ARCH

Mandibular n. 1

Facial n. 2

Glossopharyngeal n. 3

Superior laryngeal branch of vagus n. 4

Arch 5 disappears early

Recurrent laryngeal branch of vagus n. 6

Ophthalmic nerve

Optic vesicle

Maxillary nerve

BASIC STRUCTURE OF
A PHARYNGEAL ARCH

Endoderm   Ectoderm

Nerve:
Sensory -
Pretrematic division
Post-trematic division

Motor

Special visceral muscle

Arch cartilage

Arch artery

Closing membrane

Arch Cartilage Derivatives

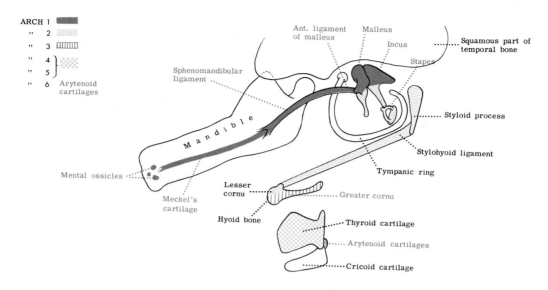

Arch cartilages and their derivatives

The condensed mesenchymal cores of the first and second arches form Meckel's and Reichert's cartilages respectively. Deep to the first ectodermal groove, however, the cores of the first and second arches and the otic vesicle all meet. In this region blastemal *auditory ossicles* develop, each being derived from more than one source. Thus the first arch derivatives are the short crus and body of the incus and the head, neck and anterior process and ligament of the malleus. The second arch derivatives are the stapes (to which the otic capsule also contributes), the long crus of the incus and the handle of the malleus. The blastemal ossicles undergo chondrification, and single ossification centres appear in each cartilage. Broadly speaking the ossicles have achieved adult size by mid-term.

Much of *Meckel's cartilage* becomes surrounded and invaded by the membranous ossification of the mandible, but between this and the anterior process and ligament of the malleus only its perichondrial sheath persists as the sphenomandibular ligament. With the incorporation of the auditory ossicles in the expanding middle-ear cavity and the ossification of the temporal bone around them, the anterior ligament of the malleus and the sphenomandibular ligament are continuous through the petrotympanic fissure. The ventral tip of Meckel's cartilage may undergo endochondral ossification, forming the mental ossicles which are later incorporated into the mandible.

Reichert's cartilage forms the styloid process, the stylohyoid ligament and the lesser cornu and upper part of the body of the hyoid bone. The third arch cartilage forms the rest of the hyoid bone. The succeeding cartilages form the larynx but the precise fate of individual cartilages is uncertain.

Special visceral (branchial) muscles

During subsequent development many of the arch muscles migrate widely from their site of origin, but they retain their original nerve supply. As far as they are known, the muscles derived from the various arches and their appropriate nerve supply are summarized in the diagram. It indicates the origin of the extrinsic ocular muscles from both first arch maxillomandibular mesenchyme and premandibular (prechordal) mesenchyme. These condensations of mesenchyme have been homologized with the head cavities of lower vertebrates and regarded as modified pre-otic somites. The diagram also indicates the presumed somitic origin of the tongue muscles.

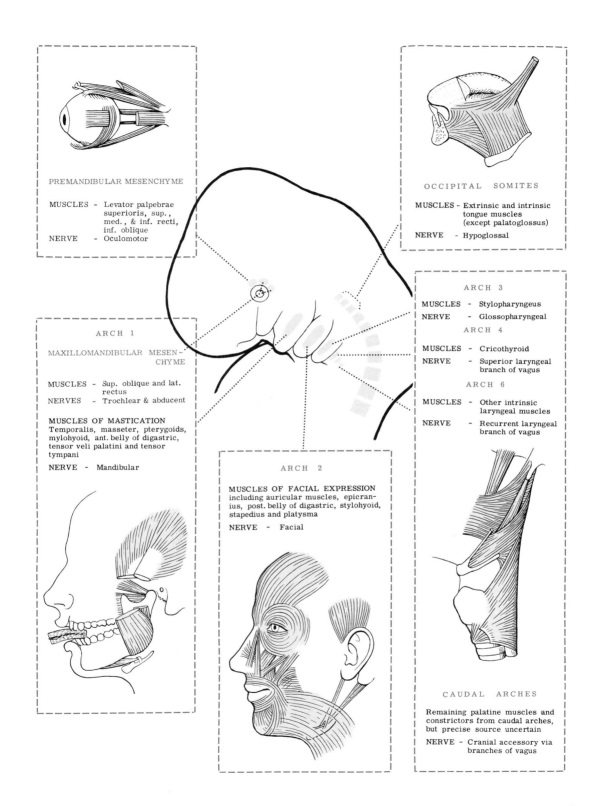

PREMANDIBULAR MESENCHYME

MUSCLES – Levator palpebrae
superioris, sup.,
med., & inf. recti,
inf. oblique
NERVE – Oculomotor

OCCIPITAL SOMITES

MUSCLES – Extrinsic and intrinsic
tongue muscles
(except palatoglossus)
NERVE – Hypoglossal

ARCH 1

MAXILLOMANDIBULAR MESEN–
CHYME

MUSCLES – Sup. oblique and lat.
rectus
NERVES – Trochlear & abducent

MUSCLES OF MASTICATION
Temporalis, masseter, pterygoids,
mylohyoid, ant. belly of digastric,
tensor veli palatini and tensor
tympani

NERVE – Mandibular

ARCH 3

MUSCLES – Stylopharyngeus
NERVE – Glossopharyngeal

ARCH 4

MUSCLES – Cricothyroid
NERVE – Superior laryngeal
branch of vagus

ARCH 6

MUSCLES – Other intrinsic
laryngeal muscles

NERVE – Recurrent laryngeal
branch of vagus

ARCH 2

MUSCLES OF FACIAL EXPRESSION
including auricular muscles, epicran-
ius, post. belly of digastric, stylohyoid,
stapedius and platysma

NERVE – Facial

CAUDAL ARCHES

Remaining palatine muscles and
constrictors from caudal arches,
but precise source uncertain

NERVE – Cranial accessory via
branches of vagus

The pharyngeal floor

In the floor of the primitive pharynx the first and second arches are large and transversely disposed, while the later arches are successively smaller and more oblique. Proliferation of the subjacent mesenchyme gives rise to a number of endodermal elevations. A small *median tongue bud (tuberculum impar)* appears between and caudal to the mandibular prominences, each of which develops a *lingual swelling*. Caudal to these three swellings the fused ventral ends of the hyoid arches transiently occupy the midline. The third, fourth and sixth arches fail to reach the midline and abut on the large, median, *copula*. A transverse groove appears at the level of the fourth arch and divides the copula into cranial and caudal halves.

The tongue

The lingual swellings enlarge and fuse with each other and the median tongue bud to form a single anterior mass. The median tongue bud probably contributes little to the adult organ. However, since the thyroid primordium develops from an endodermal invagination immediately caudal to it, and since the upper end of the invagination persists as the *foramen caecum*, any contribution which the median tongue bud makes must lie immediately anterior to the foramen. Meanwhile the cranial half of the copula enlarges and grows forwards, covering the fused ventral ends of the hyoid arches and fusing with the anterior mass. The line of fusion is indicated in the adult tongue by the *sulcus terminalis*, which separates the oral part of the tongue (arch 1) from the pharyngeal part (mainly arch 3). It seems unlikely that hyoid arch tissue is entirely excluded from the substance of the tongue and some admixture of arch tissues probably occurs.

The *endoderm* differentiates into the stratified squamous epithelium of the tongue, the cells of the taste buds, and the parenchyma and duct-lining cells of the lingual glands. The pharyngeal *mesenchyme* forms the connective tissue framework and blood and lymphatic vessels. At the root of the tongue the mesenchyme becomes seeded with lymphocytes, resulting in the formation of lymphatic nodules (lingual tonsils). The striated musculature is derived from the tissue of *occipital myotomes* which are presumed to migrate from the side of the hindbrain, passing immediately under the ectoderm, lateral to the carotid vessels, and up into the floor of the mouth to reach the tongue. These myotomic cells are followed by their segmental motor nerves which group together as the hypoglossal nerve; its course and

serial homology with the succeeding segmental motor nerves (ventral cervical nerve roots) are thus explained. The epithelial innervation of the tongue reflects its origin from arch 1 (lingual nerve and chorda tympani) and arch 3 (glossopharyngeal nerve).

The laryngeal aditus, trachea and lungs

A median depression—the *laryngotracheal groove*—develops in the pharyngeal floor caudal to the copula. Right and left *lung buds* grow from the caudal end of the floor of the groove and its margins fuse dorsal to them to form a septum dividing the foregut into laryngotracheal and oesophageal channels. The endodermal *laryngotracheal tube* thus formed grows caudally into splanchnopleuric mesoderm. Its upper end forms the larynx and its middle part the trachea. At its divided lower end each *lung bud* has a tubular portion which forms the main bronchus, and a blind extremity which forms the bronchial tree and respiratory tissues. Each grows laterally and projects into the pleural part of the intraembryonic coelom. Each main bud gives off a ventral bud, and the right bud gives off an additional craniodorsal bud. Thus are formed the lobar bronchi and the pulmonary lobes. Subsequently many generations of divisions form the finer ramifications of the bronchial tree. This process occurs during the first trimester of pregnancy. During the second, the respiratory bronchioles are developed. In the third trimester and after birth the terminal bronchioles continue to divide, and alveoli are formed. Cells of endodermal origin line the whole system. The surrounding splanchnopleuric mesoderm forms the supporting tissue and pulmonary vasculature, which develops secondary connections with the heart and sixth arch arteries.

At first, the opening of the laryngotracheal tube is a median slit, but it becomes T-shaped by the enlargement and approximation of arytenoid swellings in the ventral ends of the sixth arches. This primitive laryngeal aditus is temporarily obliterated by the fusion of its epithelial walls but becomes patent again early in the fetal period. The caudal half of the copula forms the epiglottis (and cuneiform cartilages), and as the aditus enlarges it remains connected by aryepiglottic folds to the arytenoid swellings in which form the arytenoid and corniculate cartilages.

Depressions which develop around the margins of the various elevations in the pharyngeal floor define their limits more clearly. A sulcus forms around the tongue, epiglottic valleculae form between the epiglottis and tongue, and piriform fossae form lateral to the aryepiglottic folds. From precisely which arches the thyroid and cricoid cartilages are derived remains uncertain.

The Tongue and Larynx

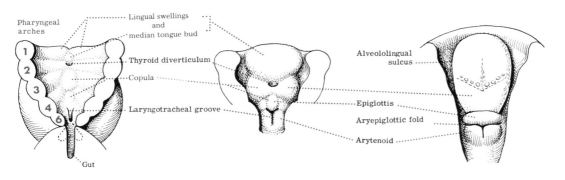

Pharyngeal arches

Lingual swellings and median tongue bud

Thyroid diverticulum

Copula

Laryngotracheal groove

Gut

Alveololingual sulcus

Epiglottis

Aryepiglottic fold

Arytenoid

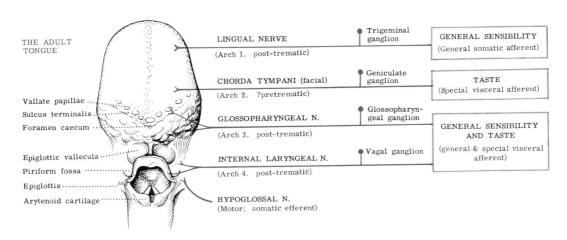

THE ADULT TONGUE

Vallate papillae

Sulcus terminalis

Foramen caecum

Epiglottic vallecula

Piriform fossa

Epiglottis

Arytenoid cartilage

LINGUAL NERVE
(Arch 1. post-trematic)

Trigeminal ganglion

GENERAL SENSIBILITY
(General somatic afferent)

CHORDA TYMPANI (facial)
(Arch 2. ?pretrematic)

Geniculate ganglion

TASTE
(Special visceral afferent)

GLOSSOPHARYNGEAL N.
(Arch 3. post-trematic)

Glossopharyn-geal ganglion

GENERAL SENSIBILITY
AND TASTE
(general & special visceral afferent)

INTERNAL LARYNGEAL N.
(Arch 4. post-trematic)

Vagal ganglion

HYPOGLOSSAL N.
(Motor; somatic efferent)

The Lungs and Bronchi

A bifurcating diverticulum develops from the ventral wall of the pharynx —

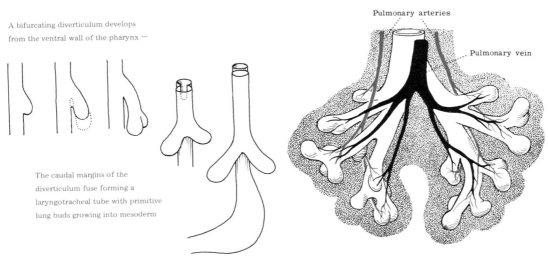

The caudal margins of the diverticulum fuse forming a laryngotracheal tube with primitive lung buds growing into mesoderm

Pulmonary arteries

Pulmonary vein

Pharyngeal pouches and endocrine glands

An early pharyngeal pouch is a simple endodermal depression between adjoining pharyngeal arches. Initially it communicates widely with the pharynx. The communication soon narrows, however, and each of pouches 2, 3 and 4 develops a *dorsal* and a *ventral recess*. The presence of the tongue prevents the development of a ventral recess in the first pouch. From the ventral recess of the fourth pouch a diverticulum—the *ultimobranchial body*—grows caudally. Sometimes it develops a transient lateral recess which approaches the ectoderm and represents the fifth pouch. This system of cavities (pouch 4, the ultimobranchial body, and pouch 5 if present) is termed the *caudal pharyngeal complex*. The whole complex communicates with the pharynx via a common duct.

On each side the dorsal recesses of the first and second pouches expand and coalesce to form a common *tubotympanic recess* with a single, narrow, pharyngeal opening. The recess approaches the ectoderm of the first groove and forms the middle-ear cavity, including the mastoid antrum and air cells, and the auditory tube.

The palatine tonsil

The ventral recess of each second pouch, between the soft palate and the tongue, forms the *palatine tonsil*. Solid endodermal cords invade the underlying mesenchyme, and central degeneration within the cords gives the system of tonsillar crypts. The intratonsillar cleft is also a remnant of the cavity of the second pouch. The mesenchyme in the intervals between the cellular cords becomes seeded with lymphocytes resulting in the formation of lymphatic nodules.

The thymus

The right and left ventral recesses of the third pouches are converted into two solid flask-shaped masses by proliferation of endodermal cells. The masses grow medially and come into contact, and form the basis of the bilobed thymus gland. The thymus lies immediately ventral to the aortic sac and, as the heart descends, follows it into the thorax. The endodermal masses are invaded by strands of mesenchyme which differentiate into the thymic blood vessels. Colony-forming units (p. 148) reach the thymus via the bloodstream and become T lymphocyte progenitors. These in their turn supply immunologically competent T lymphocytes to the general lymphatic tissues of the body via the bloodstream. The reticular cells and the concentric corpuscles of the thymus are derived from endodermal cells. Prominent in the newborn, the thymus grows in childhood, decreasing in relative size but reaching its greatest absolute size at puberty, after which it undergoes involution.

The parathyroid glands

The dorsal recess of each third pouch becomes solid by proliferation and forms a parathyroid gland. It migrates caudally with the thymus and forms an inferior parathyroid gland of the adult.

The dorsal recess of each fourth pouch forms a superior parathyroid gland. It migrates medially, with the rest of the caudal pharyngeal complex, and becomes intimately associated with the lateral aspect of the developing thyroid gland. Thymic tissue at this site may develop from the ventral recess of the fourth pharyngeal pouch. The rest of the caudal pharyngeal complex is enveloped by the developing thyroid gland and largely degenerates. However, some cells of neural crest origin persist as the calcitonin-secreting parafollicular or C cells of the thyroid gland.

The thyroid gland

A midline endodermal thickening caudal to the median tongue bud invaginates and forms a bilobed structure. It migrates caudally in the midline, ventral to the aortic sac and laryngotracheal tube, to reach its definitive position. Here it associates with the caudal pharyngeal complexes, which may possibly contribute to the gland. A hollow cellular cord—the *thyroglossal duct*—marks this path of migration. It soon degenerates but its lingual point of origin is indicated by the foramen caecum. The endodermal cells of the gland become arranged in vesicular masses—the *primary thyroid follicles*—from which generations of *secondary follicles* arise by budding. In this, as in all other glands, the connective tissue, vasculature and lymphatics develop from surrounding mesenchyme.

The suprarenal gland

The *cortex* is formed by the proliferation of cells derived from the mesoderm of the coelomic mesothelium between the primitive kidney and the root of the mesentery in the caudal half of the thoracic region. The *medulla* is formed by the migration of cells derived from the ectoderm of the spinal neural crest. These sympathochromaffin cells come into association with proliferating mesodermal tissue via developing sympathetic ganglia.

After vascularization and encapsulation by surrounding mesoderm, nests of proliferating cells under the capsule form the primitive glomerular zone. From them cords grow centripetally to constitute the *fetal cortex*, which is bulky and responsible for the relatively large size of the suprarenal in the newborn.

The fetal cortex shrinks rapidly after birth as the cords degenerate and are replaced by a definitive fascicular zone growing from the glomerular zone. The medulla is fully developed by the end of the second year but the zone remains ill-defined until puberty.

Endoderm
of Pharynx

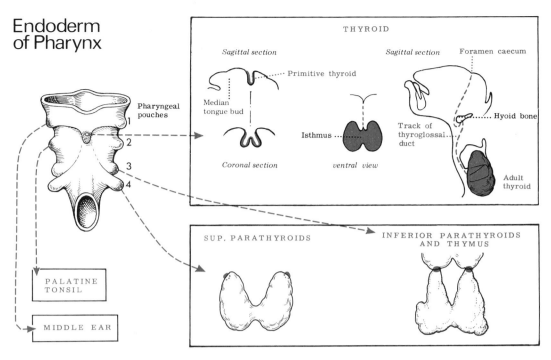

Pharyngeal
pouches

1
2
3
4

PALATINE
TONSIL

MIDDLE EAR

THYROID

Sagittal section

Primitive thyroid

Median
tongue bud

Isthmus

Coronal section

ventral view

Sagittal section

Foramen caecum

Hyoid bone

Track of
thyroglossal
duct

Adult
thyroid

SUP. PARATHYROIDS

INFERIOR PARATHYROIDS
AND THYMUS

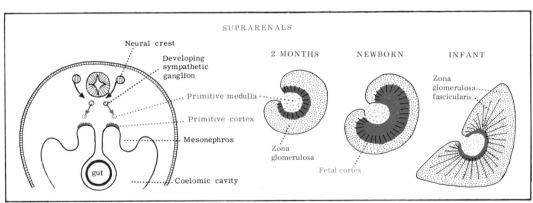

SUPRARENALS

Neural crest

Developing
sympathetic
ganglion

Primitive medulla

Primitive cortex

Mesonephros

gut

Coelomic cavity

2 MONTHS

NEWBORN

INFANT

Zona
glomerulosa

Zona
glomerulosa.
fascicularis

Fetal cortex

Anomalies

The critical processes in the development of the face and pharynx are fusion of facial prominences and palatal processes, obliteration of pharyngeal clefts and pouches, partitioning of the trachea from the oesophagus, and positional changes of the thyroid gland and the thymus.

Cleft lip, with or without cleft palate, and *cleft palate* alone are amongst the commonest congenital malformations. Whilst mutant genes, chromosomal aberrations or specific teratogens may occasionally be involved, most cases of both bear the hallmarks of polygenic inheritance. However, they are quite distinct conditions.

Cleft lip (inappropriately called 'hare lip') begins on the face and extends *backwards* for varying distances, is due to defective fusion between the maxillary and premaxillary prominences (the nasal fin and primitive palate formation may be involved) and is commoner in boys. In the most severe cases, the palatal processes are held apart and the cleft extends into the palate beyond the incisive fossa.

Cleft palate begins at the uvula and extends *forwards* for varying distances, is due to defective fusion between the palatal processes and is commoner in girls.

Oblique facial cleft may result from defective fusion between the maxillary and frontonasal prominences. Rarely, deficiency of tissue or failure of fusion results in midline anomalies such as *median cleft lip* (true hare lip), *cleft nose* and *cleft lower jaw* (of which cleft chin is a minor relatively common form).

Micrognathia—underdevelopment of the lower jaw—may be associated with tongue swallowing which can cause respiratory obstruction. *Choanal atresia* (Gk *a tretos* = not perforated) may result from failure of the oronasal membranes to break down and is also a cause of choking and of cyanosis on feeding in the newborn. A third and more common cause is a *tracheo-oesophageal fistula* (L. = tube) in which the partitioning between the air and food passages is incomplete. It is usually associated with *oesophageal atresia* which, if proximal to the fistula, results in excessive unswallowed saliva.

The only common anomalies of the lungs are those of lobes and segments.

A pharyngeal groove or pouch may persist and form a *lateral cervical (branchial) cyst* or blind-ended *sinus*, or a closing membrane may break down and form a fistulous connection between the pharynx and the skin of the neck. External cysts or openings are usually close to the anterior border of the sternomastoid muscle whilst internal openings are usually near the tonsil. The commoner *pre-auricular sinus* probably represents a persistent furrow between the tubercles which fuse to form the pinna.

Not uncommonly, part of the thyroglossal duct persists and becomes a *thyroglossal cyst*, which may rupture and form a fistula in the midline of the neck. Rarely, the thyroid gland fails to descend into the neck and remains related to the tongue (*lingual thyroid*). Variations in the form and size of the thyroid gland and of the number and location of parathyroid glands in relation to it and the thymus frequently occur. Accessory suprarenal glands, usually without medullary tissue, are also common.

CLEFT LIP

may be UNILATERAL OR BILATERAL

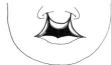
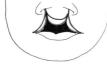

OBLIQUE FACIAL CLEFT

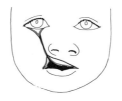

MEDIAN DEFECTS

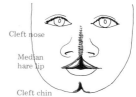

Cleft nose

Median
hare lip

Cleft chin

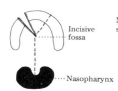

Incisive
fossa

Nasal
septum

Nasopharynx

CLEFT
PALATE

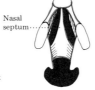

PRE-AURICULAR and LATERAL CERVICAL SINUSES AND FISTULAE

EXTERNAL OPENINGS

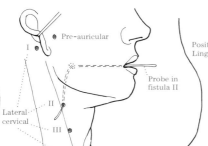

Pre-auricular

I

II

III

IV

Lateral
cervical

Probe in
fistula II

INTERNAL OPENINGS

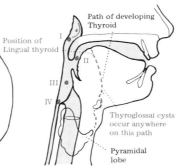

Position of
Lingual thyroid

Path of developing
Thyroid

I

II

III

IV

Thyroglossal cysts
occur anywhere
on this path

Pyramidal
lobe

MICROGNATHIA

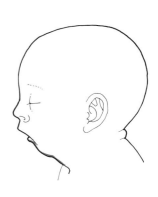

OESOPHAGEAL ATRESIA

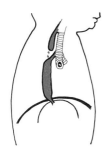
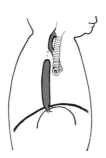
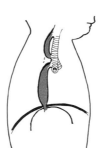
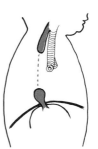

The Coelom and Gut

In development and in functional activity some organs (*viscera*) change in size, in shape and in position relative to one another and to the body wall (*soma*). This they can do more easily because of a lubricated body cavity or intraembryonic coelom between and around them.

The intraembryonic coelom, like other cavities in early development, brings nutrient fluids into direct contact with embryonic tissues and has an absorptive lining. This mechanism for absorption is not sufficient for a large and complex body, and the gut or digestive tube becomes specialized for the purpose. The large quantities of nutrients and water necessary for survival mean that the absorptive surface of the gut must also be very large. In man the absorptive surface area of its lining is increased some eleven times by folds and finger-like processes or villi. However, the area is also increased by growth, particularly in length, as a result of which the gut becomes coiled within its part of the coelom—the *peritoneal cavity*. The peritoneal cavity is then necessary for the movements and distension of the gut associated with the digestive process.

The intraembryonic coelom is first seen as a series of splits which develop in the mesoderm in front of the oral membrane and down either side of the embryo before head-fold formation. The splits coalesce to form a single U-shaped mesoderm-lined cavity which communicates with the extraembryonic coelom at the side of the embryonic disc. Nutrient fluids can then penetrate deeply between the layers of the embryo and be used by growing tissues.

With head-fold formation the limbs of the U curve down behind the pharynx and several parts of the coelom can be recognized. A midline part lies below and behind the foregut: it will form the *pericardial cavity* and the heart will grow into it. Intermediate parts lie below and to the side of the foregut: they will form the *pleural cavities* and the lungs will grow into them. The single complex *peritoneal (abdominal) cavity* forms as the parts which lie on either side of the foregut lead back and, at the umbilicus, communicate with each other and with the extraembryonic coelom.

The mesoderm lining the coelom forms smooth, shiny, lubricated membranes (*pericardium, pleura* and *peritoneum*) so that the organs can slip over each other as they grow and function. Mesoderm also forms the muscular wall of the gut but its lining is derived from endoderm.

As the heart and lungs grow and expand their respective parts of the coelom, the tissues between them seal off the pericardial from the pleural cavities. Similarly, as the liver and lungs grow, the tissues between them separate the peritoneal from the pleural cavities on each side and form part of the *diaphragm*.

At this stage the gut elongates and soon there is not enough room in the peritoneal cavity for it and the relatively large liver and kidneys which are developing there. As a result the midgut loop is extruded into the extraembryonic coelom in the base of the umbilical cord and forms the so-called *physiological hernia*. As the relative size of the liver and kidneys decreases and the size of the cavity grows, the hernia is reduced and the midgut loop returns to the abdomen. In the process the gut twists around and the order of return to the abdomen is responsible for the final layout of the large and small intestines.

The foregut, midgut and hindgut comprise a continuous tube but the parts which form from each can be recognized by the arteries which supply them. In addition to the pharynx and laryngotracheal tube, the *foregut* forms the oesophagus, the stomach and one-third of the duodenum.

From its junction with the midgut, endodermal diverticula grow into the surrounding connective tissue and form the parenchyma of the liver and pancreas. The *midgut* forms (and its artery supplies) the rest of the small bowel and over one-third of the large bowel.

The rest of the large bowel and part of the urogenital system are formed from the *hindgut*. After tail-fold formation the allantois leads from the hindgut into the umbilical cord. A spur of tissue grows from the angle between the allantois and hindgut towards the cloacal membrane and forms a septum which separates the rectum on the one hand from the bladder and urethra on the other. After the cloacal membrane has ruptured, the continuous tube of the alimentary system is open at both ends and gut endoderm and surface ectoderm meet in the anal canal as they do in the oral cavity.

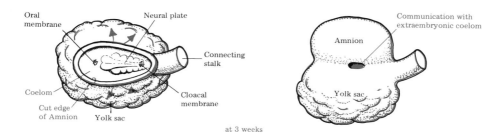

Oral membrane

Neural plate

Connecting stalk

Coelom

Cut edge of Amnion

Yolk sac

Cloacal membrane

at 3 weeks

Communication with extraembryonic coelom

Amnion

Yolk sac

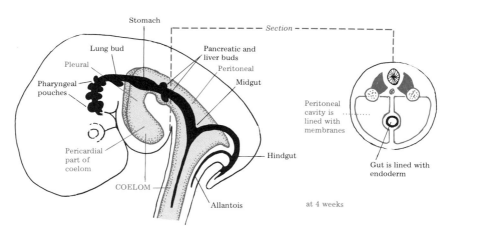

Stomach

Lung bud

Pleural

Pharyngeal pouches

Pericardial part of coelom

COELOM

Section

Pancreatic and liver buds

Peritoneal

Midgut

Hindgut

Allantois

Peritoneal cavity is lined with membranes

Gut is lined with endoderm

at 4 weeks

The coelom

The primitive *intraembryonic coelom* forms by the coalescence of multiple clefts which appear in lateral plate mesoderm and in the cardiogenic area and septum transversum. At first the horseshoe-shaped cavity is closed and, caudally, its limbs end blindly. Cranially, they are continuous across the midline in the future pericardial region. The junctional zone of mesoderm alongside the caudal blind ends has, until this stage, separated the intraembryonic coelom from the extraembryonic coelom but it breaks down. Each limb of the intraembryonic coelom is then in wide communication with the extraembryonic coelom and provides an indirect connection between it and the primitive pericardial cavity. With head-fold formation, the pericardial region and septum transversum swing ventrally and then caudally to include a part of the yolk sac within the embryo as the foregut. With tail-fold formation, part of the yolk sac is included within the embryo as the hindgut. Since the allantoic diverticulum grows from this part of the yolk sac, its base is also drawn into the embryo. With the allantois comes the angle of junction between the yolk sac and the connecting stalk, so that a part of the coelom, originally extraembryonic, is drawn into the body. With lateral-fold formation, the wide communications between the limbs of the intraembryonic coelom and the extraembryonic coelom swing on to the ventral aspect of the embryo. The caudal margins of these communications may temporarily be separated from each other by mesoderm in the angle of junction between the allantois and yolk sac. As this is drawn into the body with tail-fold formation, the communications become continuous with each other across the midline, between the allantois and the stalk of the yolk sac. The general arrangement of the coelom at the end of fold formation is shown well in transverse sections and in relation to the outline of a late somite embryo on p. 57.

Illustrations opposite show coeloms of slightly older embryos after removal of the surrounding tissues. The midline *pericardial cavity* lies ventral to the foregut and communicates with the *peritoneal cavity* via a pair of *pleuroperitoneal canals* which flank the foregut and its derivatives. These canals are separate bilateral cavities, with the foregut between them. The midgut and hindgut, however, are co-extensive with the communications between the intraembryonic and the extraembryonic coelom; ventral to these parts of the gut the two sides of the coelom are continuous across the midline. With expansion of the peritoneal cavity and narrowing of the umbilicus, the communication between the intra- and extraembryonic coelom is progressively restricted and is finally obliterated as the umbilical cord consolidates. However, a cavity, into which a *physiological hernia of the midgut* later occurs, remains in the base of the cord.

The developing lung buds project into the medial aspect of the pleuroperitoneal canals and define a pair of primitive *pleural cavities*. These remain continuous with the pericardial and peritoneal cavities via pleuropericardial and pleuroperitoneal openings respectively. The *pleuropericardial opening* on each side is encircled by the phrenic nerve and the common cardinal vein. As the lungs and pleural cavities enlarge lateral to these structures, and the heart and pericardial cavity cranial to them, they become isolated in the free edge of a *pleuropericardial membrane*. This eventually fuses with pre-oesophageal mesoderm and cuts off the pericardial cavity from the pleural cavities. The latter extend into the ventral wall of the pericardial cavity, and split it into superficial (body wall) and deep (parietal pericardial) layers. They continue to extend ventrally until the pleural cavities are separated by only a narrow strip of mesoderm which forms the sternopericardial ligaments. Thus are explained the deep position of the parietal pericardium (a somatopleuric layer) and the position of the phrenic nerves and the derivatives of the common cardinal veins, medial to the lungs and pleural sacs.

The lungs also extend downwards and strip mesoderm off the lateral body wall, between them and the liver, forming a *pleuroperitoneal membrane* on each side. This projects into the lateral aspect of the *pleuroperitoneal opening* and eventually fuses with the septum transversum ventral to the foregut and with the mesoderm (*dorsal mesogastrium*) dorsal to it. Thus, a mesodermal *diaphragm*, separating the pleural and peritoneal cavities, is formed. Further extension of the pleural cavities into the dorsal and lateral body wall adds peripheral contributions to the diaphragm, but the extent of these and other contributions is not certainly known. The early diaphragm is sited ventral to the cervical spinal cord and is invaded by muscle tissue derived mainly from the fourth cervical myotomes. The final position of the diaphragm is reached only after elongation of the neck, descent of the heart and expansion of the pericardial and pleural cavities. Thus is explained the apparently curious origin and course of the phrenic nerve.

The Coelom

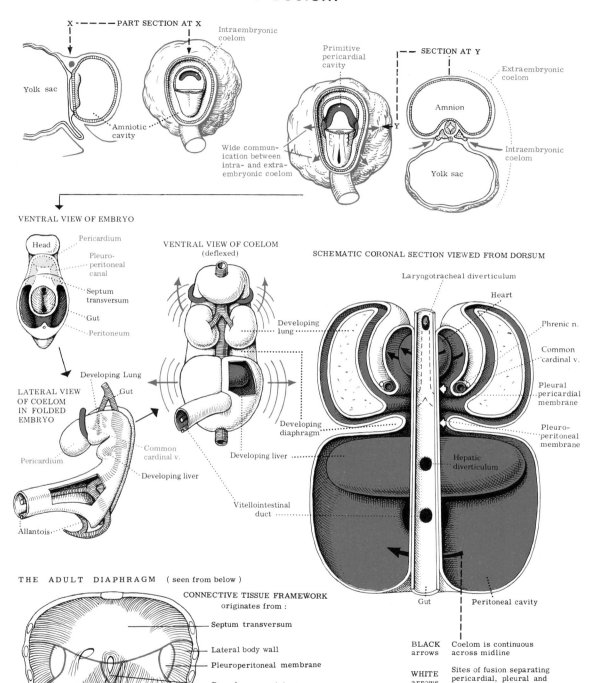

PART SECTION AT X

Intraembryonic coelom

Yolk sac

Amniotic cavity

Primitive pericardial cavity

SECTION AT Y

Extraembryonic coelom

Amnion

Intraembryonic coelom

Wide communication between intra- and extra-embryonic coelom

Yolk sac

VENTRAL VIEW OF EMBRYO

Head

Pericardium

Pleuro-peritoneal canal

Septum transversum

Gut

Peritoneum

VENTRAL VIEW OF COELOM (deflexed)

Developing lung

Developing diaphragm

Developing liver

Vitellointestinal duct

LATERAL VIEW OF COELOM IN FOLDED EMBRYO

Developing Lung

Gut

Pericardium

Common cardinal v.

Developing liver

Allantois

SCHEMATIC CORONAL SECTION VIEWED FROM DORSUM

Laryngotracheal diverticulum

Heart

Phrenic n.

Common cardinal v.

Pleural pericardial membrane

Pleuro-peritoneal membrane

Hepatic diverticulum

Gut

Peritoneal cavity

THE ADULT DIAPHRAGM (seen from below)

CONNECTIVE TISSUE FRAMEWORK originates from :

Septum transversum

Lateral body wall

Pleuroperitoneal membrane

Dorsal mesogastrium

Dorsal body wall

BLACK arrows — Coelom is continuous across midline

WHITE arrows — Sites of fusion separating pericardial, pleural and peritoneal cavities

MUSCLE originates chiefly from the 4th cervical myotomes

Gut, peritoneum, pancreas and liver

With the descent of the heart and diaphragm, the part of the foregut between the pharynx and diaphragm elongates rapidly to form the *oesophagus*. The elongation is accompanied by epithelial proliferation with virtual obliteration of its lumen, followed by recanalization and differentiation of a stratified squamous epithelium. This part of the endodermal gut tube is embedded in lateral plate mesoderm which forms striated muscle cranially, grading into smooth muscle caudally.

The remainder of the foregut forms the *stomach* and the *duodenum*, as far as the opening of the bile duct. Whereas the cranial part of the septum transversum contributes to the ventral part of the diaphragm, its caudal part forms a partition—the *ventral mesogastrium*—ventral to these parts of the foregut. The primitive *stomach* soon assumes a characteristic shape as it develops a lesser curvature, continuous with the ventral mesogastrium, and a greater curvature, continuous with its dorsal mesentery (mesogastrium). Growth changes in the stomach and adjacent liver, and cavitation in the surrounding mesoderm, cause the stomach to rotate so that its greater curvature comes to lie on the left. The original left surface is now ventral—hence the definitive ventral surface of the stomach is supplied mainly by the left vagus nerve. With the rotation of the stomach the *duodenum* is carried to the right. It makes contact with the dorsal parietal peritoneum and fuses with it, largely losing its mesentery and becoming retroperitoneal.

Before the stomach rotates, the *ventral mesogastrium* is a thick midline mesodermal partition extending from the lesser curvature of the stomach to the diaphragm and ventral body wall and having a free caudal margin extending to the umbilicus. The developing liver and biliary passages grow into this ventral mesogastrium from the duodenum and divide it into various regions. That part between the lesser curvature of the stomach and the dorsal aspect of the liver is the future *lesser omentum*. Its free border contains the bile duct, hepatic artery and portal vein and they enter the liver at the porta hepatis. The next part of the ventral mesogastrium contributes to the substance of the *liver* and forms its peritoneal investment. That part between the liver and the diaphragm and ventral abdominal wall is the future *falciform ligament*. Its free border carries the left umbilical vein to the liver. As the lobes of the liver and coelomic recesses develop, the peritoneal reflections of the liver become more complex.

The *pancreas* arises from two endodermal diverticula—dorsal and ventral—which grow out from the duodenal wall into the surrounding mesenchyme. The *dorsal diverticulum* arises a little cranial to the level of the hepatic diverticulum but the *ventral diverticulum* arises in common with it. Cellular cords, which divide repeatedly, arise from both diverticula. The tips of some cords remain solid, separate from the rest of the cord, and differentiate into endocrine islet tissue. The remainder of the cords canalize, and their endodermal cells differentiate into exocrine pancreatic cells. The original diverticula and their main branches form the duct systems of the pancreas, while the surrounding mesenchyme forms the scanty connective tissue, capillaries and lymphatics. As the stomach and duodenum rotate, growth changes in the duodenal wall cause the ventral pancreas and the common hepatopancreatic orifice to migrate around the dorsal (originally right) wall of the duodenum until the concavity of the duodenal loop is reached. Fusion between the dorsal and ventral pancreas then occurs and their duct systems intercommunicate. The ventral rudiment forms the lower part of the head of the pancreas. Its duct, which continues to open into the duodenum with the bile duct (hepatic diverticulum), persists. The dorsal rudiment forms the rest of the pancreas and the greater part of its duct joins the ventral duct, together forming the main pancreatic duct. The remainder of the dorsal duct forms an accessory pancreatic duct which drains the upper part of the head and may have a separate small opening into the duodenum, cranial to the hepatopancreatic ampulla.

The *dorsal mesogastrium* is originally attached to the midline of the dorsal abdominal wall but, after the stomach rotates, its line of attachment shifts and in general follows the contour of the greater curvature. The spleen develops as a circumscribed thickening of the dorsal mesogastrium which enlarges and projects from its left surface. Local mesoderm forms the capsule, connective tissues and vasculature of the spleen but it is seeded by colony-forming units and lymphocytes which form transitory haemopoietic and definitive lymphoid tissues (p. 148).

The early foregut mesenteries are thick mesodermal masses and, in association with rotation of the stomach, they become excavated by a series of recesses. From the right side of the stomach a *pneumato-enteric recess* excavates, dorsal to the liver, towards the right lung bud. The cranial part of this recess is isolated by the closure of the pleuroperitoneal opening as the infracardiac bursa; the caudal part shares a common entrance with a *pancreaticoenteric recess* which excavates from right to left behind the stomach and thins and expands the greater omentum. A *hepatoenteric recess* thins and expands the lesser omentum.

The early *omental bursa* (lesser sac) is formed by the expansion and confluence of these recesses during rotation of the stomach. With rotation, the plane of the lesser omentum changes from sagittal to coronal, and the parietal attachment of the *dorsal mesogastrium* also changes. Its attachment now sweeps from the oesophageal orifice downwards and to the left across the diaphragm and the upper pole of the left kidney and then veers to the right across the dorsal abdominal wall to reach the first part of the duodenum. The various parts of the dorsal mesogastrium may

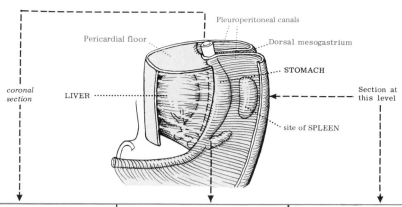

Pleuroperitoneal canals
Pericardial floor
Dorsal mesogastrium
STOMACH
LIVER
Section at this level
coronal section
site of SPLEEN

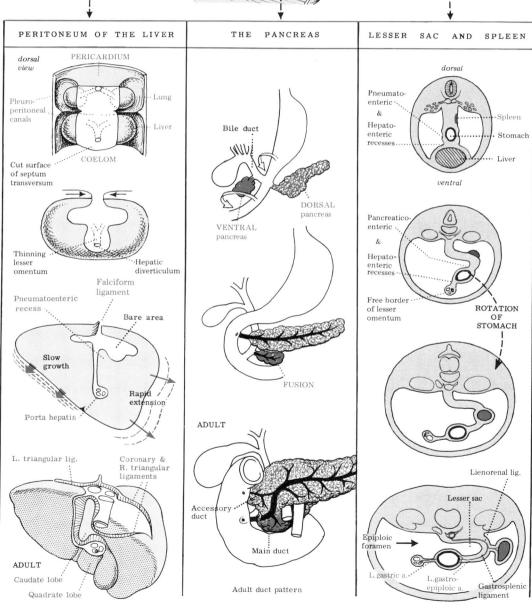

PERITONEUM OF THE LIVER	THE PANCREAS	LESSER SAC AND SPLEEN

PERITONEUM OF THE LIVER

dorsal view

PERICARDIUM

Pleuro-peritoneal canals

Lung

Liver

COELOM

Cut surface of septum transversum

Thinning lesser omentum

Hepatic diverticulum

Pneumatoenteric recess

Falciform ligament

Bare area

Slow growth

Porta hepatis

Rapid extension

L. triangular lig.

Coronary & R. triangular ligaments

ADULT

Caudate lobe

Quadrate lobe

THE PANCREAS

Bile duct

DORSAL pancreas

VENTRAL pancreas

FUSION

ADULT

Accessory duct

Main duct

Adult duct pattern

LESSER SAC AND SPLEEN

dorsal

Pneumato-enteric & Hepato-enteric recesses

Spleen

Stomach

Liver

ventral

Pancreatico-enteric & Hepato-enteric recesses

Free border of lesser omentum

ROTATION OF STOMACH

Lienorenal lig.

Lesser sac

Epiploic foramen

L.gastric a.

L.gastro-epiploic a.

Gastrosplenic ligament

87

now be designated—the *gastrophrenic, gastrosplenic (gastrolienal)* and *lienorenal ligaments* and the *greater omentum*. The greater omentum pouches more and more over midgut and hindgut derivatives to form the characteristic apron-like double fold of dorsal mesogastrium. The omental bursa then lies dorsal to the lesser omentum, the stomach and the gastrosplenic and gastrophrenic ligaments. Its *inferior recess*, which is derived from the pancreaticoenteric recess, passes down for a variable distance between the layers of the greater omentum. It also passes up into a *superior recess* which is derived from hepatoenteric and the subdiaphragmatic part of the right pneumatoenteric recesses and has the caudate lobe of the liver projecting into it. As the duodenum becomes retroperitoneal, the aditus to the lesser sac—the *epiploic foramen*—becomes narrow, relative to surrounding structures. Its definitive boundaries are the caudate process of the liver, the posterior parietal peritoneum, the first part of the duodenum and the free border of the lesser omentum with its contained structures.

The midgut forms the *duodenum* (beyond the hepatopancreatic ampulla), the *jejunum*, the *ileum*, the *caecum*, the *appendix*, the *ascending colon* and the right two-thirds of the *transverse colon*. The primitive midgut forms a loop, the apex of which is continuous with the narrowing stalk of the yolk sac. The midgut loop elongates rapidly and, at the same time, the liver and primitive kidneys enlarge and almost fill the abdominal cavity. As a result the midgut and an elongated dorsal mesentery are extruded into the extraembryonic coelom which persists in the umbilical cord. This extrusion constitutes the *physiological hernia of the midgut*. While in the hernial sac the proximal limb of the midgut further elongates, coils and comes to occupy the right side of the sac. This and subsequent examples of dextral asymmetry probably result from directional viscous drag produced by ciliary action of coelomic epithelium. The distal limb grows much less rapidly, occupies the left side of the sac and develops a diverticulum—the *primitive caecum*—with a conical appendix as its apex.

Return of the midgut to the abdomen occurs in the third month and accompanies a relative decrease in the size of the liver and primitive kidneys. The proximal limb (small bowel) re-enters first and passes to the right of the hindgut and its mesentery, and dorsal to the superior mesenteric artery. The future descending colon is thus displaced to the left and the distal limb of the midgut loop is drawn out of the hernial sac. The caecum and appendix are the last structures to return to the abdomen and come to lie low in the right iliac fossa. The proximal colon then runs transversely across the abdomen below the liver to join the hindgut, which turns up and over the small bowel at the splenic flexure. The hindgut continues as the descending colon which descends vertically on the left, the sigmoid colon which curves medially and the rectum which descends in the midline. As the lower border of the liver rises in the abdomen, the proximal colon becomes oblique and then angulated into ascending and transverse parts, the last crossing the duodenum and the transverse mesocolon adhering to it.

As parts of the gut successively reach relatively definitive positions their mesenteric attachments undergo modification. Mesenteries may shorten, their attachments may move and organs may become more or less retroperitoneal by fusion and disappearance of peritoneal layers (*zygosis*). A similar process occurs as the greater omentum pouches downwards and forwards over the transverse colon and its mesocolon. Fusion occurs between the visceral peritoneum of the transverse colon and the upper layer of the transverse mesocolon on the one hand, and the posterior (returning) layer of the greater omentum, on the other. The main blood vessels of the gut tube and its derivatives (p. 154) follow the planes of its mesenteries and do not cross planes of fusion. At birth the appendix still forms the apex of the caecum. After birth differential growth occurs and the appendix migrates on the posteromedial wall of the caecum.

The hindgut forms the left third of the *transverse colon*, the *descending colon*, the *sigmoid colon*, the *rectum*, the upper part of the *anal canal* and certain *urogenital organs*. The separation of the last from the primitive rectum is effected by the *urorectal septum* which grows from the angle between the allantois and hindgut towards the cloacal membrane (p. 94). The caudal end of the urorectal septum forms the primitive *perineal body*. The anal canal is completed by a somatopleuric component. Anal swellings encircle the canal (p. 98) and their ectodermal covering is continuous with the endodermal lining of the hindgut at the site of the ruptured cloacal membrane. This lies somewhat below the so-called anal valves. The different developmental origins of the upper and lower anal canal are reflected in their different epithelia, nerve supply, arterial blood supply, venous drainage and lymphatic drainage.

The histogenesis of the intestines

The splanchnopleuric wall of the early gut tube consists of a lining of endodermal cells, an external covering of flattened visceral mesodermal cells, which are part of the general lining of the intraembryonic coelom, and an intervening thick layer of loose visceral mesenchyme. The endodermal cells form the gut epithelium and, by tubular prolongations into the overlying mesenchyme, the secretory and duct-lining cells of the intestinal glands. Most digestive enzymes are present by mid-pregnancy but amylase appears after birth. The external flattened cells form the visceral peritoneum. The intervening mesenchyme forms the blood vessels, lymphatics, connective tissue framework and smooth muscle of the intestinal wall and is seeded with lymphocytes to form solitary and aggregate lymphatic nodules.

Gut and Mesenteries

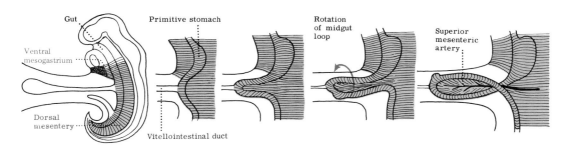

Gut
Ventral mesogastrium
Dorsal mesentery
Primitive stomach
Vitellointestinal duct
Rotation of midgut loop
Superior mesenteric artery

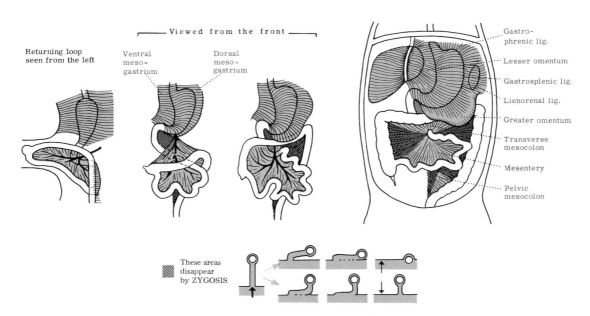

Returning loop seen from the left

— Viewed from the front —

Ventral meso-gastrium
Dorsal meso-gastrium

Gastro-phrenic lig.
Lesser omentum
Gastrosplenic lig.
Lienorenal lig.
Greater omentum
Transverse mesocolon
Mesentery
Pelvic mesocolon

These areas disappear by ZYGOSIS

The retroperitoneal organs and lines of peritoneal reflection after final fixation of the gut

The adult mesenteries in sagittal section

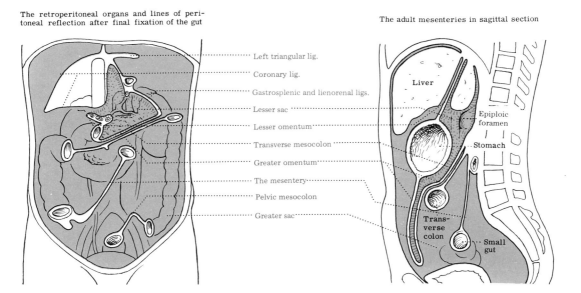

Left triangular lig.
Coronary lig.
Gastrosplenic and lienorenal ligs.
Lesser sac
Lesser omentum
Transverse mesocolon
Greater omentum
The mesentery
Pelvic mesocolon
Greater sac

Liver
Epiploic foramen
Stomach
Transverse colon
Small gut

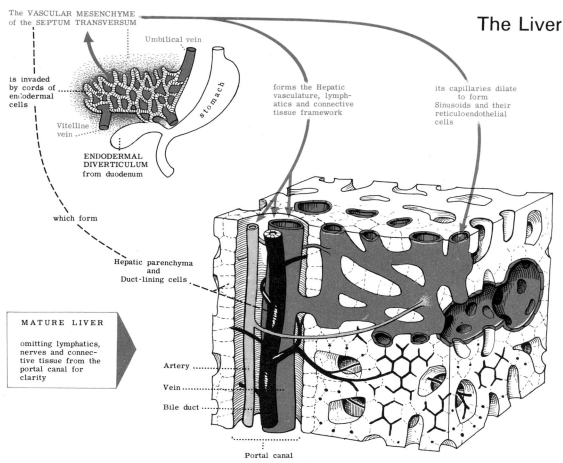

The VASCULAR MESENCHYME
of the SEPTUM TRANSVERSUM

is invaded
by cords of
endodermal
cells

Umbilical vein

stomach

Vitelline
vein

ENDODERMAL
DIVERTICULUM
from duodenum

forms the Hepatic
vasculature, lymph-
atics and connective
tissue framework

its capillaries dilate
to form
Sinusoids and their
reticuloendothelial
cells

which form

Hepatic parenchyma
and
Duct-lining cells

MATURE LIVER

omitting lymphatics,
nerves and connec-
tive tissue from the
portal canal for
clarity

Artery

Vein

Bile duct

Portal canal

The hepatic rudiment appears in somite embryos as a thickening of the endoderm in the angle between the foregut and yolk sac. As the duodenum forms, the *hepatic diverticulum* arises from this thickening and grows into the mesoderm of the septum transversum (ventral mesogastrium). The mesoderm is permeated by a capillary plexus which caudally receives the vitelline and umbilical veins, and cranially drains into the heart via the hepatocardiac veins (p. 156). The apex of the endodermal diverticulum divides into *right* and *left hepatic buds,* from which solid cylinders of endodermal cells grow into the vascular mesoderm. The cylinders continually subdivide and anastomose, forming a spongework of endodermal cells with intervening vascular mesenchyme which, having been seeded with colony-forming units (p. 148), becomes the principal site of haemopoiesis. A further solid bud, the primordium of the *gall bladder,* arises from the original stem. It is usually said that stem and buds canalize from the gut end to form the bile duct, hepatic ducts, bile capillaries and gall bladder. However, there is some evidence that the duct system originates in the liver as certain parenchyma cells become surrounded by mesenchyme and differentiate into duct-lining cells. The intrahepatic

lumina then connect up with each other and canalization spreads throughout the duct system from the hepatic end. Whatever their mode of origin, the right and left hepatic ducts drain right and left developmental lobes which do not correspond to the lobes of descriptive anatomy. The left lobe, developmentally and functionally, includes the whole of the quadrate lobe and half of the caudate lobe.

Anomalies

Stenosis (Gk *stenos* = narrow) or *atresia* of the gut lumen most commonly occur at sites where epithelial proliferation is a feature of normal development—i.e. the oesophagus, the duodenum, the upper jejunum, the lower ileum, the colon and the rectum.

In the case of the oesophagus, atresia may be associated with anomalous partitioning between the laryngotracheal and gut tubes resulting in a *tracheo-oesophageal fistula* (p. 81), most commonly below the atresia. In several conditions gastric mucosa may be found in thoracic gut: rarely, the oesophagus may fail to elongate sufficiently, resulting in a *congenital short oesophagus with thoracic stomach,* partial or complete; more commonly, abnormal epithelial differentiation

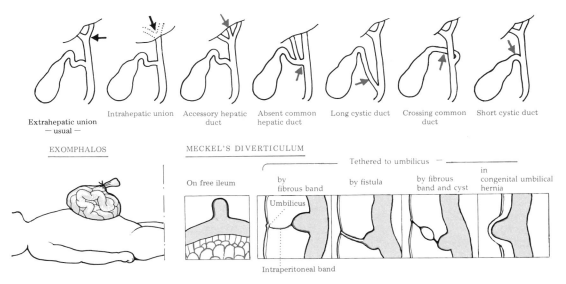

Extrahepatic union — usual —

Intrahepatic union

Accessory hepatic duct

Absent common hepatic duct

Long cystic duct

Crossing common duct

Short cystic duct

EXOMPHALOS

MECKEL'S DIVERTICULUM

Tethered to umbilicus

On free ileum

by fibrous band

by fistula

by fibrous band and cyst

in congenital umbilical hernia

Umbilicus

Intraperitoneal band

results in *heterotopic* (Gk *heteros topos* = other place) *gastric mucosa* in the oesophagus; the commonest cause is *oesophageal hiatus hernia* in which the abnormally large hiatus (L. = opening) is congenital but the herniation of the stomach is acquired and rarely manifests itself before adulthood. On the other hand, *posterolateral defects of the diaphragm*, in which a pleuroperitoneal opening remains patent, are most frequently found in infancy: the defect is usually on the left side and the thorax contains small intestine but not uncommonly contains colon, stomach and spleen as well. Their presence may inhibit development and inflation of the lungs.

Abnormal epithelial differentiation is responsible for the only common truly congenital anomaly of the stomach—*heterotopic pancreatic mucosa*—an anomaly also commonly found in the duodenum. So-called congenital but more correctly called *infantile pyloric stenosis* is not present from birth but develops in the neonatal period. This very common condition occurs predominantly in males (5:1) and bears the hallmarks of multifactorial inheritance. Anomalous lobes or segments of the liver are rare but variations (other than atresia) of the hepatic, cystic and common bile ducts (including their vascularization) and of the pancreatic ducts are common.

Non-rotation or *malrotation of the gut* may result in bizarre positioning of the viscera with highly atypical mesenteries. *Anomalous peritoneal folds* commonly occur and are often associated with defective fixation of the duodenum, of the ascending or of the descending colon. The caecum may rise from the iliac fossa with the liver—*subhepatic* caecum. Occasionally, a terminal, conical, *infantile appendix* persists. The physiological hernia of the midgut may not return to the abdomen so that, at birth, coils of intestine are found outside a very large umbilicus in a thin-walled

sac derived from the amnion—a condition called *exomphalos*. This is distinct from *congenital umbilical hernia* in which the midgut loop has returned to the abdomen but the umbilicus has not closed so that there is a slight protrusion through it which is covered by skin.

The stalk of the yolk sac may persist in various forms: Meckel's diverticulum occurs on the antimesenteric border of the ileum about a metre proximal to the caecum and frequently contains *heterotopic gastric mucosa; a cyst, fibrous cord* or *fistula* may connect the bowel and umbilicus; the umbilical end of the duct may persist as a blind-ended *sinus*.

The urorectal septum may not partition the cloaca completely, resulting in a *fistula* connecting the rectum with either the bladder, the urethra, the vagina or the perineum (p. 101). This may be associated with *atresia* of the terminal gut which may then end above the pelvic diaphragm—*anorectal atresia*—or below it— *anal atresia*. Rarely, the anal membrane fails to break down—*membranous atresia*.

In *situs inversus* the bilateral asymmetry of the viscera is reversed. Organs normally found on the left side, such as the stomach and spleen, are sited on the right side and vice versa. The thoracic viscera may also be involved. The condition may be due to an autosomal recessive gene and be associated with the *immotile cilia syndrome* in which all cilia including spermatozoa and embryonic cilia are affected. Normal embryonic ciliary action is believed to produce directional viscous drag which results in dextral asymmetry in early embryogenesis. In the absence of ciliary activity, asymmetry is random and 50 per cent of cases of *immotile cilia syndrome* have *situs inversus*. Sporadic incomplete examples may be due to the deflexion of looped structures by abnormal local pressures.

The Urogenital System

The function of the urinary system is to maintain the internal environment of the body by adjusting the composition of the blood. First the blood is filtered but then essential water, salt and glucose are returned to it while surplus water and the end products of metabolism are conveyed in the urine to the exterior (p. 9). The function of the genital system is to produce gametes and to deliver them to the site of fertilization (p. 32). Although their functions are quite distinct, they are closely linked in development. They have their origin in mesoderm, which projects into the peritoneal cavity and is *intermediate* in position between the mesoderm lining it and the *paraxial mesoderm* which lies alongside the notochord.

Secretory tubules which develop in the *intermediate mesoderm* of the thoracic and lumbar regions form a temporary kidney or *mesonephros* on each side. The tubules open into the *Wolffian duct*, which leads to the *cloaca*. A bud, which will form the ureter and collecting system, grows from the cloacal end of the Wolffian duct into the intermediate mesoderm of the sacral region where the secretory tubules of the definitive kidney (*metanephros*) develop. After the cloaca is partitioned into the rectum on the one hand and the bladder and urethra on the other, the ureters open into the bladder and elongate as the kidneys 'rise' into the lumbar region.

Even before the mesonephros ceases to function as a urinary organ, the genital system begins to develop within it. The epithelium on its lateral side turns in and encloses the *Müllerian duct* which grows caudally. At first it grows alongside the Wolffian duct but then crosses it to meet the Müllerian duct of the other side and reach the cloaca in the midline. The medial part of the mesonephros is invaded by primordial sex cells and bulges into the peritoneal cavity as a gonad. Although sex was determined at the time of fertilization (p. 15), the gonads and ducts of the two sexes are indistinguishable at this stage. The *external genitalia*, too, are similar. In both sexes a groove leads from the under-surface of a *phallus* back between *genital folds* and *swellings*.

In the male, gonads soon develop the structure of *testes* and begin to secrete male sex hormones which affect both the ducts associated with the mesonephros and the external genitalia. As a result, the *Wolffian duct* on each side is taken over as a genital duct and forms the ductus (vas) deferens and the ejaculatory duct which convey sperms from the testis to the urethra; the Müllerian ducts degenerate. Under the influence of male sex hormones the phallus forms the penis, the *genital folds fuse* to enclose the penile urethra while the *genital swellings fuse* to form the scrotum into which the testes descend.

In the female, the gonads develop the structure of *ovaries* and begin to secrete female sex hormones. However, it is the absence of male sex hormones which affects the ducts and external genitalia. As a result, the *Müllerian ducts* form the uterine tubes and the uterus in which fertilization and implantation, respectively, occur; the Wolffian ducts degenerate. Again, in the absence of male sex hormones the phallus remains small and forms the clitoris and the *genital folds and swellings remain unfused* and form the labia on either side of the introitus.

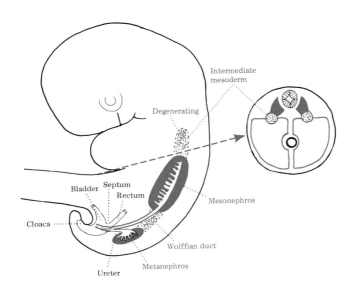

Intermediate mesoderm

Degenerating

Bladder
Septum
Rectum

Cloaca

Mesonephros

Wolffian duct

Ureter

Metanephros

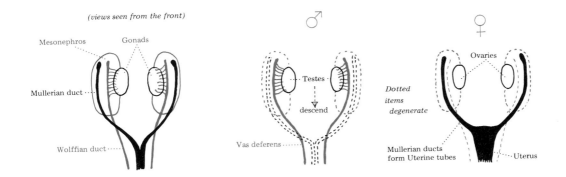

(views seen from the front)

♂

♀

Mesonephros

Gonads

Mullerian duct

Wolffian duct

Testes

descend

Vas deferens

Ovaries

Dotted items degenerate

Mullerian ducts form Uterine tubes

Uterus

EXTERNAL GENITALIA

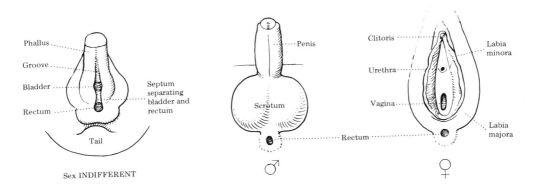

Phallus

Groove

Bladder

Rectum

Septum separating bladder and rectum

Tail

Sex INDIFFERENT

Penis

Scrotum

Rectum

♂

Clitoris

Urethra

Vagina

Labia minora

Labia majora

Rectum

♀

93

Kidneys and bladder

The development of the excretory system in most lower vertebrates (e.g. cyclostomes) is summarized in the diagram. A similar *pronephros* is found in the more cranial segments of larval Anamniotes but is succeeded in the adult by a larger, more caudal and more complex *mesonephros*.

In man there is no true pronephros but some segmental cavitation and rudimentary tubule formation occurs in the intermediate mesoderm opposite the cervical somites. The remainder of the intermediate mesoderm forms an unsegmented *nephrogenic cord*. From its dorsal part the *nephric duct* develops as a solid rod of cells which separates from the nephrogenic cord, grows back to reach the lateral wall of the cloaca and then canalizes from the cranial end. Under the influence of the nephric duct, clusters of cells in the cranial part of the nephrogenic cord form vesicles which elongate to become *mesonephric tubules*. The lateral end of each tubule reaches and taps the nephric (*Wolffian*) duct. The intermediate part becomes S-shaped. The medial end expands and is invaginated by a *glomerulus*. Tubule formation progresses caudally until, at the height of its development, the mesonephros is a spindle-shaped ridge projecting into the coelom and extending from the septum transversum to the third lumbar segment. After functioning for a limited period, degeneration overtakes the tubules in the more cranial segments, leaving only those of the lumbar region, which persist in connection with the genital system.

The metanephros

Meanwhile, a hollow *ureteric bud* arises from the Wolffian duct near its cloacal end. It grows dorsally and cranially into the sacral region of the nephrogenic cord, where it induces the formation of a *metanephric cap*. In its turn the metanephric cap induces the dilated tip of the ureteric bud to divide and give rise to two or three future major calyces. These, in their turn, give rise to minor calyces and so on until some 13 generations of divisions (*tubules*) are present. The metanephric tissue proliferates and divides with the ureteric bud so that each branch tubule has its own cap. The tubules of the third and fourth generations are subsequently absorbed into the minor calyces, which thus receive those of the fifth generation as the papillary ducts of Bellini. Later generations form the collecting tubules. The metanephric cap on the end of each tubule is induced to become vesicular and then S-shaped, with one extremity tapping the collecting tubule and the other being invaginated by a glomerular tuft. Thus the secretory and collecting tubules are developmentally and functionally distinct.

The first few generations of secretory tubules, nearest the medulla, are only temporary structures. Later generations are induced progressively as collecting tubules extend into the cortex. These more peripheral nephrons are grouped and give the fetal kidney its characteristic lobulated appearance which may be related to its segmentation. During development the kidney 'ascends' about four segments. This apparent migration is due to growth of the lumbar and sacral regions of the body and to straightening of its curvature, and is accompanied by growth and elongation of the ureter. As the kidney 'ascends' it is vascularized by successively higher lateral splanchnic arteries until it reaches the caudal pole of the suprarenal gland and shares its definitive blood supply. The fetal kidney is functional from mid-term and urine is passed into the amniotic cavity where, together with lung secretions, it replenishes the liquor amnii.

The bladder

Caudal growth of the *urorectal septum*, the wedge of tissue between the allantois and hindgut, has meanwhile divided the cloaca into a dorsal rectum, and a *ventral part* which is demarcated into *primitive bladder* and *urogenital sinus* by the openings of the Wolffian ducts. The caudal part of these ducts is absorbed into the bladder so that the ureters and ducts come to have separate openings in its dorsal wall. At first, the openings of the Wolffian ducts are cranial to those of the ureters, but with differential growth and absorption the ureteric openings migrate laterally and the Wolffian openings migrate caudally between them. The ureteric openings form the lateral angles, and the near-midline Wolffian openings the caudal angle, of the future *trigone*. Thus, in contrast to the rest of the bladder, the epithelium of the trigone is derived from mesoderm. It may later be overgrown by surrounding epithelium so that the definitive lining of the bladder is wholly endodermal in origin. The apex of the bladder tapers to form the *urachus*, which is continuous at the umbilicus with the degenerating allantois. The bladder and urachus elongate proportionately as the infraumbilical abdominal wall forms. After birth the urachus forms a fibrous cord—the median umbilical ligament—within which a cavity, continuous with that of the bladder, persists for about one-third of its length.

Excretory System of Lower Vertebrate

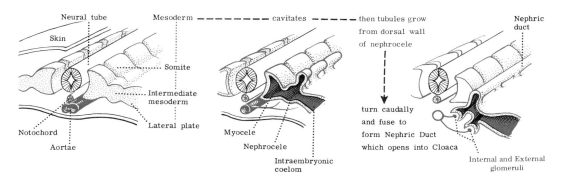

Neural tube
Skin
Somite
Intermediate mesoderm
Lateral plate
Notochord
Aortae

Mesoderm ———— cavitates ———— then tubules grow from dorsal wall of nephrocele

Myocele
Nephrocele
Intraembryonic coelom

turn caudally and fuse to form Nephric Duct which opens into Cloaca

Nephric duct

Internal and External glomeruli

Human Nephric System

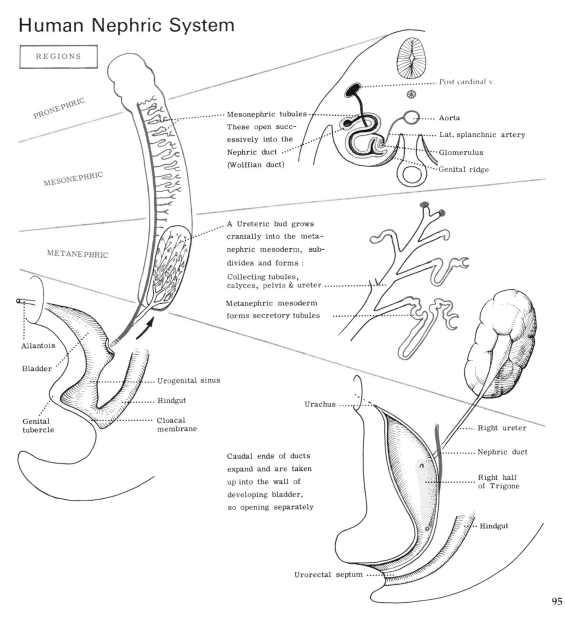

REGIONS

PRONEPHRIC

MESONEPHRIC

METANEPHRIC

Mesonephric tubules
These open successively into the
Nephric duct
(Wolffian duct)

Post cardinal v.
Aorta
Lat. splanchnic artery
Glomerulus
Genital ridge

A Ureteric bud grows cranially into the metanephric mesoderm, subdivides and forms :
Collecting tubules, calyces, pelvis & ureter
Metanephric mesoderm forms secretory tubules

Allantois
Bladder
Genital tubercle

Urogenital sinus
Hindgut
Cloacal membrane

Caudal ends of ducts expand and are taken up into the wall of developing bladder, so opening separately

Urachus
Right ureter
Nephric duct
Right half of Trigone
Hindgut

Urorectal septum

Gonads and ducts

Primordial sex cells probably arise from epiblast and pass through the primitive streak with mesoderm destined for the yolk sac. In the presomite human embryo they can be recognized in relation to yolk sac endoderm caudal to the embryonic disc. Tail-fold formation carries the multiplying cells into the wall of the hindgut whence they migrate via the dorsal mesentery to lie in and beneath the epithelium on the medial aspect of the mesonephros. They induce the epithelium to proliferate so that it bulges into the coelom as a *genital ridge*. Soon the epithelium loses its basement membrane and ill-defined cellular cords penetrate the underlying mesenchyme. As these carry the primordial sex cells with them they are known as *sex cords*. At this stage, the gonads are histologically indifferent. Although chromosomal sex was determined at the time of fertilization, and may be identified by a chromatin test on the cells, histodifferentiation of the sexes has not yet occurred. On the lateral aspect of each mesonephros, near its cranial end, an invagination of coelomic epithelium forms a *Müllerian (paramesonephric) duct* which grows caudally. The Müllerian duct at first courses lateral to the Wolffian duct, but more caudally crosses its ventral aspect to meet the Müllerian duct of the opposite side. The two Müllerian ducts then run longitudinally to end blindly on the dorsal wall of the urogenital sinus, between the Wolffian ducts, where they produce an elevation termed the *Müllerian tubercle.*

In the male

The differentiation of gonads into testes seems to depend largely upon the action of a cell membrane antigen (H–Y). The regulator gene for H–Y synthesis is borne on the Y chromosome but genes on the X chromosome and on autosomes are also involved in male differentiation (in all at least 19 genes are involved).

Secretions of fetal testes (androgens, Wolffian stabilizer and Müllerian repressor) are responsible for the differentiation of male ducts and external genitalia.

The testis is first recognizable as such when mesenchyme spreads beneath the surface epithelium and between the sex cords as the future *tunica albuginea* and its septa. The peripheral parts of the sex cords enlarge, split into daughter cords and form *seminiferous tubules*. The primordial sex cells form spermatogonia and the supporting cord cells form the cells of Sertoli. The central parts of the sex cords converge and fuse to form the *rete testis*. The testis is invaded by mesenchyme cells of mesonephric origin, some of which persist as interstitial cells. The rete connects with the glomerular ends of some six to twelve persisting mesonephric tubules which thus form the *efferent ductules* and lobules of the epididymis. In this way the *Wolffian duct* becomes the *male genital duct* and forms the duct of the epididymis, the ductus deferens and, near the Müllerian tubercle, the ejaculatory duct. The terminal part of the ductus deferens dilates to form the ampulla near which the seminal vesicle arises as a diverticulum. The Müllerian tubercle forms the seminal colliculus while an endodermal vaginal plate (cf. female) forms the prostatic utricle. Most of the Müllerian duct degenerates, but its cranial tip and that of the Wolffian duct persist as the appendages of the testis and epididymis respectively. Persisting mesonephric tubules form the paradidymis and aberrant ductules.

In the female

In H–Y-negative individuals, differentiation of the gonads occurs later than in males. The sex cords

Development of the Gonads

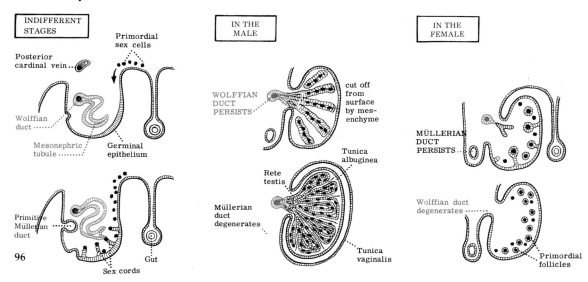

INDIFFERENT STAGES

Primordial sex cells

Posterior cardinal vein

Wolffian duct

Mesonephric tubule

Germinal epithelium

Primitive Müllerian duct

Gut

Sex cords

IN THE MALE

WOLFFIAN DUCT PERSISTS

cut off from surface by mesenchyme

Tunica albuginea

Rete testis

Müllerian duct degenerates

Tunica vaginalis

IN THE FEMALE

MÜLLERIAN DUCT PERSISTS

Wolffian duct degenerates

Primordial follicles

converge to form a primitive rete but do not become isolated from the coelomic epithelium by a tunica albuginea. Within them primordial sex cells form oogonia, and they and their surrounding epithelial cells, derived from coelomic epithelium, divide repeatedly. Mesenchyme breaks up the sex cords and forms the ovarian stroma. Oogonia progressively enter meiosis and are arrested in its early stages as primary oocytes. The epithelial cells surrounding them form the pregranulosa cells of primordial follicles. The number of germ cells peak at about 7 million at mid-term but atresia is already well under way so that, of the 2 million remaining at term, about 1 million are atretic.

In the absence of stimuli from fetal testes, the *Müllerian ducts* form most of the *female genital tract*. On each side, the cranial longitudinal part forms the uterine tube and its coelomic opening develops fimbriae. The caudal longitudinal parts fuse and form the cervix uteri. The intermediate unfused parts of the ducts expand, coalesce and are incorporated into the uterus as the fundus and the body.

At first, the caudal blind end of the fused ducts (future external os) is at the Müllerian tubercle (site of future hymen) but epithelial proliferation forms a *vaginal plate* which increasingly separates them. The central cells of the plate subsequently break down and form a vaginal lumen which expands cranially and caudally to delimit the vaginal fornices and the hymen respectively.

The Wolffian system persists only as functionless vestiges. The cranial end of the Wolffian duct forms vesicular appendages. Its intermediate part, together with those mesonephric tubules which connected up with the rete ovarii, persists as the duct and tubules of the epoophoron which lies between the layers of the broad ligament. More caudal tubules end blindly and form the paroophoron which is also in the broad ligament but between the epoophoron and the uterus. The caudal part of the Wolffian duct degenerates slowly and forms Gartner's duct, which may be traced alongside the genital tract from epoophoron to hymen.

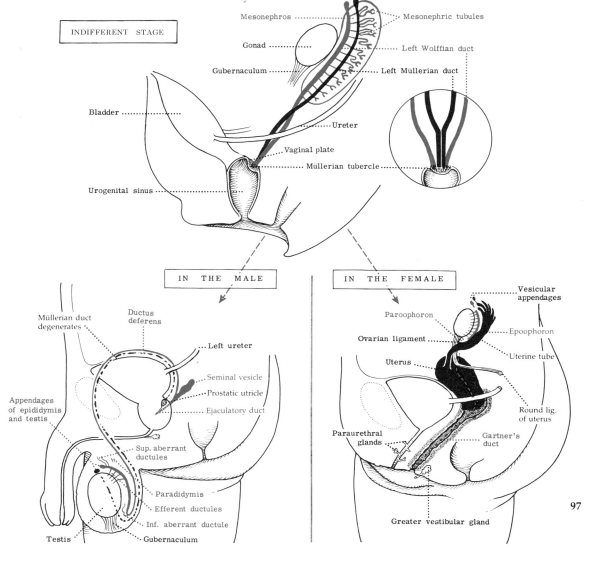

INDIFFERENT STAGE

Mesonephros ·············· Mesonephric tubules
Gonad ··········
Gubernaculum ············ Left Wolffian duct
Left Müllerian duct
Bladder ·········
Ureter
Vaginal plate
Müllerian tubercle ··········
Urogenital sinus ·················

IN THE MALE

Müllerian duct degenerates ··
Ductus deferens
Left ureter
Seminal vesicle
Prostatic utricle
Ejaculatory duct
Appendages of epididymis and testis
Sup. aberrant ductules
Paradidymis
Efferent ductules
Inf. aberrant ductule
Testis   Gubernaculum

IN THE FEMALE

Paroophoron
Vesicular appendages
Ovarian ligament ··········
Epoophoron
Uterus ·········
Uterine tube
Round lig. of uterus
Paraurethral glands ···········
Gartner's duct
Greater vestibular gland

97

External genitalia

After tail-fold formation the *cloacal membrane* lies in a depression between the umbilicus and the primitive streak, from which proliferating mesoderm streams in all directions. Two major streams flank the cloacal membrane. They raise *lateral swellings* on either side of it and form a *genital tubercle* cranial to it. Beyond the genital tubercle they form the matrix of the infraumbilical abdominal wall. The genital tubercle elongates as a *phallus* and the *urogenital sinus* extends into its base. Here the endodermal sinus epithelium proliferates and forms a *urethral plate* which grows towards the tip of the phallus. Meanwhile the cloacal depression extends on to the caudal aspect of the phallus as a *urethral groove* and is bounded by *genital folds* distinct from the lateral swellings. The ectoderm of the floor of the urethral groove is in contact with the endoderm of the urethral plate. As the urorectal septum reaches it, the cloacal membrane breaks down. The breakdown process extends into the floor of the urethral groove, deepens it and exposes the endodermal urethral plate. The leading edge of the urorectal septum (future perineal body) is then covered by ingrowth of tissues from either side so that the genital folds meet immediately in front of the anus and the lateral swellings are subdivided into *genital* and *anal parts*. In both sexes the *anal swellings* gradually encircle the anal canal. Their covering ectoderm lines the anal canal as far as the site of the ruptured membrane. Beyond this it is lined with cloacal endoderm in continuity with that of the hindgut.

In the female

The *neck of the primitive bladder* elongates to form the whole of the urethra. At the same time the urogenital sinus becomes shallower, retains its perineal orifice and forms the vestibule. As a result of these changes, the Müllerian tubercle (future hymen) and the lower end of the neck of the primitive bladder (future external urinary meatus) approach the surface. The *genital folds* become the labia minora, and the *genital swellings* (the labia majora, and the *phallus*) the clitoris. Paraurethral ducts and vestibular and urethral glands arise as diverticula of the urogenital sinus.

In the male

Under the influence of dihydrotestosterone, a metabolite of testosterone, *the neck of the primitive bladder* forms the prostatic urethra as far as the utricle where the Müllerian tubercle becomes the seminal colliculus. The glandular part of the prostate develops from five groups of outgrowths from this region corresponding to the definitive lobes. Smooth muscle differentiates from the surrounding mesenchyme. Beyond the prostatic utricle, the *pelvic part of the urogenital sinus* forms the rest of the prostatic urethra and the membranous urethra. As the *genital folds* close over the phallic part of the sinus and the urethral groove, from behind forwards, the urogenital orifice migrates along the ventral aspect of the phallus. The *genital swellings* also come together and fuse to form the scrotum. Meanwhile the phallus has

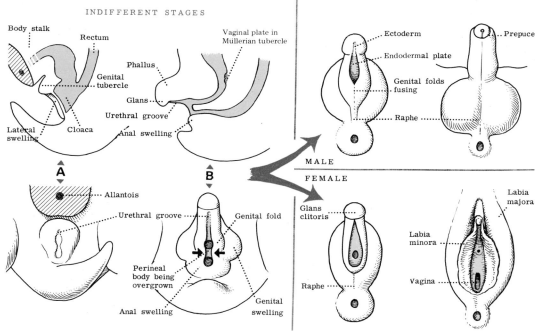

INDIFFERENT STAGES

enlarged to become the penis, and ectoderm has grown in from its tip (glans) to meet the urethral plate. This ectoderm also becomes exposed as the breakdown process extends along the urethral groove. Fusion of the genital folds results in a spongy urethra lined mainly with endoderm but with ectoderm in the glans. A fold of skin from the base of the glans grows over and adheres to it. This *prepuce* remains partially adherent until 6 months or more after birth. Bulbourethral and urethral glands arise as diverticula of the phallic part of the urogenital sinus.

Descent of the gonads

The caudal end of the developing gonad remains in continuity with the mesonephros. Near the crossing of the Müllerian and Wolffian ducts the mesonephric ridge is connected to the inguinal region by a peritoneal fold. A column of mesenchyme—the *gubernaculum*—differentiates in this peritoneal inguinal fold and leads from the *gonad* into the *genital swelling*. The abdominal muscles subsequently develop around the gubernaculum and form the inguinal canal. In both sexes the gonads undergo a relative shift caudally. The factors concerned include degeneration of the

mesonephros and cranial end of the gonad and rapid growth of the body wall. The gonad thus 'descends' some ten segments but retains its neurovascular supply from the higher level. It projects into the inguinal fossa of peritoneum, from which a diverticulum—the *processus vaginalis*—extends down the inguinal canal, ventral to the gubernaculum.

In the male, the testis remains near the deep inguinal ring for some months. Given the appropriate hormonal stimulus-response, it then quickly descends the inguinal canal and normally reaches the scrotum in the month before birth. The surrounding part of the processus persists as the tunica vaginalis, the remainder being obliterated at, or soon after, birth. The coverings of the spermatic cord differentiate from the mesenchyme of the gubernaculum.

In the female, the gubernaculum becomes secondarily attached to the cornu of the uterus forming the ovarian ligament proximal to it and the round ligament distal to it. The processus vaginalis is normally obliterated before birth. The ovary remains in the false pelvis until the pelvic basin deepens during childhood, when it descends with the other pelvic viscera. Its long axis remains vertical in the nulliparous woman.

Ascent of Kidneys and Descent of Gonads

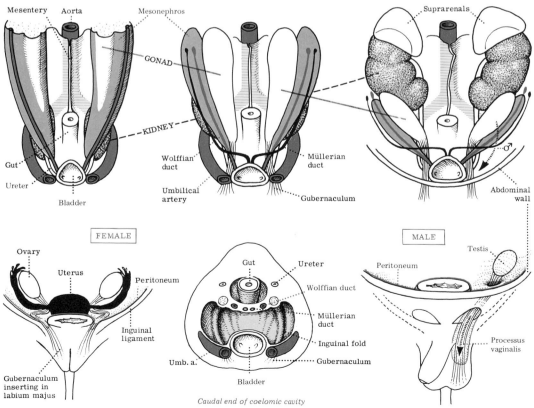

Caudal end of coelomic cavity

Anomalies

Unilateral renal agenesis or *hypoplasia*, which are common conditions, result from failure of the ureteric bud to induce tubule formation in the metanephros. In *bilateral renal agenesis*, which is uncommon and incompatible with life, anuria produces oligohydramnios and thus other deformities, including the compression facies (p. 168). Cysts occur in the kidney more frequently than in any other organ: some are attributable to failure of the collecting and secretory tubules to unite; others to persistence of vestigial tubules. *Congenital polycystic kidney* occurs in infantile non-familial and adult familial (autosomal) forms. *Double pelvis and ureter* result from branching of the ureteric bud. Ectopia of one kidney is common and results from its failure to 'ascend', usually remaining in the pelvis. In *horseshoe kidney* right and left primordia have fused at their lower poles; in general the more extensive the fusion the less the kidney 'ascends' from the pelvis.

The urachus may persist in various forms: commonly a *urachal diverticulum* opens from the bladder while a *urachal cyst* occurs between it and the umbilicus; a *urachal sinus* opening at the umbilicus is much less common and a *congenital patent urachus* is very rare.

Ectopic ureteral orifices, which are often associated with double ureter, may open into the bladder outside the trigone, into the urethra, into a seminal vesicle or into the vestibule or vagina.

Stenosis or *atresia* most commonly occur at sites where epithelial proliferation is a feature of normal development: *stenosis of a ureteral orifice* may produce a *ureterocele*—a ballooning of the lower end of the ureter into the bladder; *posterior urethral valves* occur in the region of the seminal colliculus; atresia *of the anterior urethra* and particularly *meatal stenosis* are common. Less common are the conditions of *hypospadias* and *epispadias*, although the latter occurs more frequently with *exstrophy of the bladder*.

Anomalies of the male reproductive ducts are uncommon but those of the female are not, *imperforate hymen* (persistence of the lower end of the vaginal plate) and *double uterus* being the commonest.

The only common gonadal anomaly is *undescended testis (cryptorchism), maldescended testis (ectopia)* and *ovarian ectopia (descended ovary)* being rare. For normal spermatogenesis the testis needs the lower and controllable temperature which is achievable in the scrotum, and a testis which is brought down before the age of 5 years may become functional.

Congenital agonadism means complete absence of functional ovarian or testicular tissue, usually with a female duct system and external genitalia. In some cases a fetal testis may have been transiently present and have produced male or intersex development.

Differentiation of the gonads depends upon the expressivity of numerous genes. Very rarely, an individual with both ovarian and testicular tissue results. *True hermaphroditism* may be bilateral with an *ovotestis* on each side, unilateral with a single ovotestis, or lateral with an ovary on one side and a testis on the other. Extragonadal differentiation varies widely, but in most lateral hermaphrodites the development of the duct system is lateral and corresponds to the gonad of that side.

In *male pseudohermaphroditism* scrotal or cryptorchid testes are present and the sex chromosome complement is normal. Hypospadias is the commonest form but many varieties of extragonadal differentiation are found. At puberty masculinization usually occurs when the external genitalia are of the male or intersex type whereas feminization occurs when they are of the female type and the interstitial cells of the testis produce large quantities of oestrogens.

In *female pseudohermaphroditism* the ovaries have a normal sex chromosome complement. Usually, female ducts are present and masculinization is restricted to the urogenital sinus and external genitalia. The commonest form has a single urogenital orifice at the vulva and a hypertrophied clitoris, but more masculine forms occur. The androgen responsible may be fetal or maternal in origin or may have been administered to the mother.

TESTICULAR DESCENT _____ may be ARRESTED (cryptorchism)

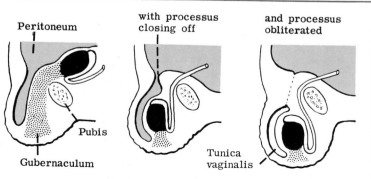

Peritoneum

with processus closing off

and processus obliterated

Pubis

Gubernaculum

Tunica vaginalis

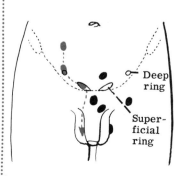

Deep ring

Super-ficial ring

If processus remains patent, abdominal contents may descend
- CONGENITAL INGUINAL HERNIA - or fluid may collect -
CONGENITAL HYDROCELE

... or may be ABERRANT

(ectopia testis)

HORSESHOE KIDNEY

Note fetal lobulation and double ureters

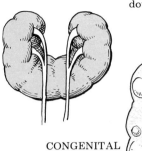

CONGENITAL POLYCYSTIC KIDNEY

HYPOSPADIAS

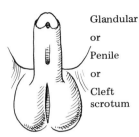

Glandular

or

Penile

or

Cleft scrotum

Genital folds fail to fuse and whole or part of urethral groove and phallic urogenital sinus persist.

EXSTROPHY OF THE BLADDER AND EPISPADIAS

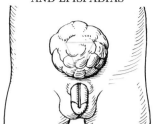

Failure of fusion of midline infra-umbilical mesoderm with separation of the pubic bones. Dorsal wall of phallus and ventral wall of abdomen and bladder fail to fuse.

ANOMALIES OF MULLERIAN DUCTS

DOUBLE UTERUS AND VAGINA

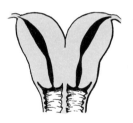

Mullerian ducts remain unfused and induce bi-lateral vaginal plates

DOUBLE UTERUS WITH DOUBLE CERVIX

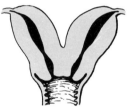

or a single vaginal plate

DOUBLE UTERUS WITH SINGLE CERVIX

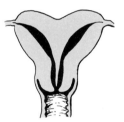

Incorporation may not occur

SEPTATE UTERUS

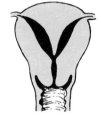

or may be incomplete

ANOMALIES OF CLOACAL REGION

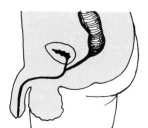

RECTOURETHRAL FISTULA

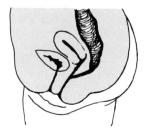

RECTOVAGINAL FISTULA

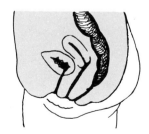

ECTOPIC ANUS

Urorectal septum fails to complete separation of rectum from urogenital sinus

Rectum ends above pelvic diaphragm (anorectal atresia) or below it (anal atresia)

Somites, Bone, Skull and Limbs

Late in the third week of development the embryo is three-layered. Occupying the midline of the middle layer is the *notochord* and, on each side, between it and the intermediate mesoderm is a continuous column of *paraxial mesoderm*. Most of the column becomes divided into short segments, each of which is called a *somite* (Gk = body segment). The formation of symmetrically paired somites begins shortly behind the oral membrane and proceeds caudally. The somites are readily seen in surface contour, and form such a conspicuous feature that the number of pairs present is used as a means of staging embryos of the fourth week (p. 64). By 4 weeks about 30 pairs have formed and they become difficult to count, and embryos are then staged by length. However, the number of somites continues to increase during the next 2 weeks until there are over 40 pairs.

From side views of embryos at this stage it might appear that the somites represent a segmented vertebral column but this is not the case. Unlike the vertebral column, the somites are not midline structures and they do not correspond in position to individual vertebrae. The notochord is the midline supporting structure at this stage and cells flow from the somites to form a continuous column of connective tissue surrounding it. The column then becomes segmented into embryonic connective tissue (*membranous* or *blastemal*) models of individual vertebrae with intervertebral discs between them. Other cells flow from the somites beneath the ectoderm to form the connective tissue layer of the skin—the *dermis*—while the ectoderm itself forms the epithelial layer—the *epidermis*.

The remaining somite cells form striated skeletal muscle fibres, some of which attach to the vertebral column and move it while others migrate into the body wall where they produce movements, including those of respiration, and where they affect intra-abdominal pressure.

Bone is essentially mineralized connective tissue. In situations such as the vault of the skull and the face, the cells on a membranous model of the future bone begin to secrete a structureless matrix around themselves. Fibrils appear in the matrix, and mineral crystals appear on, in and between them. As a result the cells become encased in bone which spreads through the membranous model, a process called *ossification in membrane*. Growth occurs at the periphery of the bone by accretion.

In other situations, such as the vertebrae and the bones of the limbs, an intermediate stage is interposed. After fibrils have appeared in the matrix, it is transformed into gristle or cartilage and the process spreads so that the *membranous model* of the future bone becomes cartilaginous. Bone forms beneath the limiting membrane of the *cartilaginous model* and within it. At centres within the cartilaginous model, cells become degenerate and the matrix becomes calcified before being eroded by vascular connective tissue. Bone is then deposited on remnants of calcified cartilage. With this intermediate stage, the process is called *ossification in cartilage*. It, too, spreads within the model but growth occurs not only at the periphery but also at the interfaces between bone and cartilage—*growth cartilages*—as both continue to form. Whether ossified in membrane or in cartilage, bones undergo remodelling as they grow. This entails a balance between the activities of bone-forming cells—*osteoblasts*—and those of bone-resorbing cells—*osteoclasts*. Bone then develops a microscopic structure in relation to the small blood vessels which pervade it and to prevailing mechanical stresses.

Whereas the vault of the skull and the bones of the face ossify in membrane and meet and grow at sutures, the base of the skull and the capsules enclosing the sense organs ossify in cartilage and have growth cartilages between them. Not all the hard tissues of the skull are derived from connective tissue. Unlike the bones, the teeth have their origin in ectoderm and form from a fascinating interaction between epithelial and connective tissues. Ectodermal buds grow into subjacent connective tissue and influence (*induce*) cells in it to become dentine-forming *odontoblasts*. Only in the presence of dentine do the epithelial cells (*ameloblasts*) form tooth enamel. This type of interaction between tissues is a common developmental mechanism.

The limbs are first seen as projections from the body wall opposite the lower cervical and lumbosacral somites. These projections gradually develop shape and internal structure (bones, muscles and blood vessels). All these form from the connective tissue of the limb bud itself but nerves grow into the limb bud from the spinal cord.

Ossification

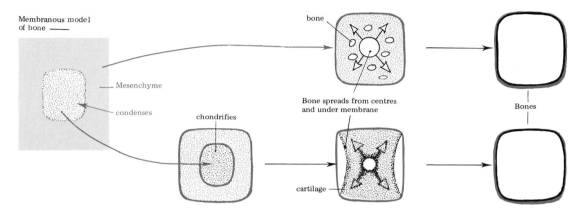

OSSIFICATION IN MEMBRANE

Membranous model
of bone

Mesenchyme

condenses

bone

Bone spreads from centres
and under membrane

chondrifies

cartilage

Bones

OSSIFICATION IN CARTILAGE

Somites and Limbs

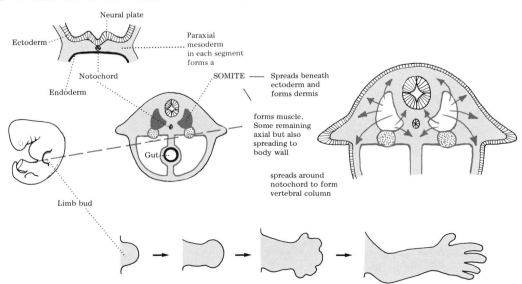

Neural plate

Ectoderm

Notochord

Endoderm

Paraxial
mesoderm
in each segment
forms a

SOMITE — Spreads beneath
ectoderm and
forms dermis

forms muscle.
Some remaining
axial but also
spreading to
body wall

Gut

spreads around
notochord to form
vertebral column

Limb bud

The somites and axial skeleton

The foundation of a metamerically segmented body is laid down when a succession of transverse crevices cuts into the paraxial mesoderm and divides it into somites. The formation and differentiation of somites begins a short distance behind the cranial tip of the notochord and extends caudally, so that there are formed, in turn, 4 occipital, 8 cervical, 12 thoracic, 5 lumbar, 5 sacral and 5–10 coccygeal pairs of somites. Of these, the first occipital and the last few coccygeal pairs are evanescent.

Initially, the epithelial cells of the somite are arranged radially round a central spherical cavity. With further growth, the cavity becomes a thin vertical slit separating outer and inner walls which correspond to the parietal and visceral layers of lateral plate mesoderm but are separated from them by the intermediate cell mass. The ventral part of the inner wall breaks up into a mass of mesenchyme cells—the *sclerotome*. The cells of the sclerotome migrate medially, envelop the notochord and contribute to the axial skeleton and meninges. Cells proliferating from the dorsal part of the inner wall of the somite form the *myotome* and give rise to somatic muscle. A segmental nerve grows out from the neural tube to each myotome. The remaining (outer) wall—the *dermatome*—becomes mesenchymatous, spreads beneath the ectoderm and contributes to the connective tissue layer of the skin and subcutaneous tissues.

The *notochord* is the primitive axial supporting structure. With the medial migration of sclerotomic tissue, it becomes encased in a continuous cylinder of mesenchyme: individual sclerotomes can then be identified only by their position in relation to somites and intersegmental vessels. In the lateral part of each cranial sclerotome-half, cells bound a *vertebral notch* around a segmental nerve. The density of cells in the lateral part of each caudal sclerotome-half increases and gives rise to dorsal and ventral outgrowths. The *dorsal outgrowth* grows back between two segmental nerves and around the neural tube to meet its fellow of the opposite side as a vertebral arch. The *ventral outgrowth* grows between two myotomes as a costal process. Meanwhile, condensation of cells around the notochord has formed an unsegmented *perichordal sheath*. Each zone of cell density spreads medially from the base of a vertebral arch to meet the perichordal sheath. The latter is then segmented by a series of *discs* of increased cell density. Adjoining *blastemal* vertebral bodies are delimited by these discs which contribute to their subsequent growth, each forming the annulus fibrosus of an intervertebral disc. Mucoid degeneration of the notochordal cells and of the inner aspect of the annulus fibrosus forms the nucleus pulposus. Between the developing discs the notochord retrogresses as two expanding centres of chondrification appear and fuse to form a cartilaginous centrum around it.

Meanwhile, there appear regional differences in the development of the costal process. In the thoracic and cervical regions an area of rarefaction, in which a longitudinal anastomosis between successive intersegmental arteries will form, develops in the root of each *blastemal* process. Separate centres of *chondrification* appear in each neural arch and in each costal process. From the former, a cartilaginous transverse process grows through the blastema, dorsal to the arterial anastomosis, to meet the latter. In the thoracic region each costal process forms a cartilaginous rib, and costotransverse and costovertebral joints are represented by mesenchymatous interzones between the cartilaginous neural arch and rib. In the cervical region each costal process remains short, and the corresponding interzones fuse. The foramen transversarium is thus bounded ventrally and laterally by the cartilaginous costal process and dorsally by the transverse process. In the lumbar and sacral regions, areas of rarefaction do not appear in the short blastemal costal processes, and the cartilaginous transverse and costal processes fuse. The subsequent *ossification* of a vertebra is represented diagrammatically. Separate costal centres are limited to the thoracic and lower cervical vertebrae.

The cells of the myotome elongate and differentiate into striated muscle fibres. At first the muscles are segmental and separated by the costal processes of blastemal vertebrae. Except in relation to the axial skeleton this segmentation is lost as myotomes migrate, fuse with each other, split up into subunits or degenerate. In this way the myotomes form the intrinsic muscles of the back, the abdominal muscles and the intercostal muscles. The remaining musculature differentiates in situ in mesenchyme of lateral plate origin (appendicular muscles) or in mixed head mesenchyme of lateral plate, neural crest, prechordal plate and somite origin (orbital, pharyngeal arch and tongue muscles).

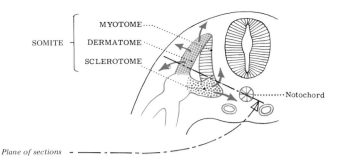

SOMITE {
MYOTOME
DERMATOME
SCLEROTOME
}

Notochord

Plane of sections

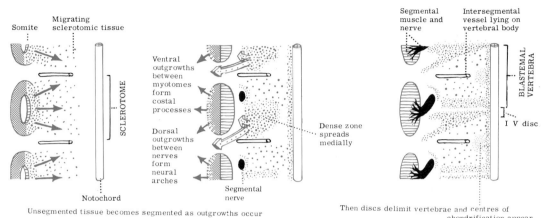

Somite

Migrating sclerotomic tissue

SCLEROTOME

Notochord

Ventral outgrowths between myotomes form costal processes

Dorsal outgrowths between nerves form neural arches

Segmental nerve

Dense zone spreads medially

Segmental muscle and nerve

Intersegmental vessel lying on vertebral body

BLASTEMAL VERTEBRA

I V disc

Unsegmented tissue becomes segmented as outgrowths occur

Then discs delimit vertebrae and centres of chondrification appear

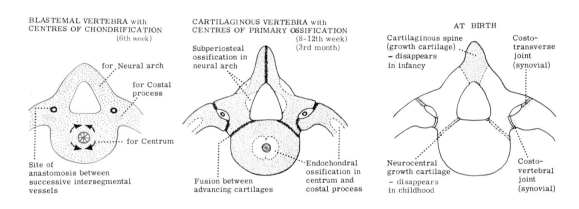

BLASTEMAL VERTEBRA with CENTRES OF CHONDRIFICATION (6th week)

for Neural arch

for Costal process

for Centrum

Site of anastomosis between successive intersegmental vessels

CARTILAGINOUS VERTEBRA with CENTRES OF PRIMARY OSSIFICATION (8-12th week) (3rd month)

Subperiosteal ossification in neural arch

Fusion between advancing cartilages

Endochondral ossification in centrum and costal process

AT BIRTH

Cartilaginous spine (growth cartilage) – disappears in infancy

Costo-transverse joint (synovial)

Neurocentral growth cartilage – disappears in childhood

Costo-vertebral joint (synovial)

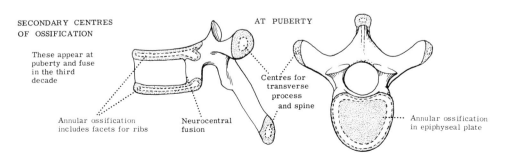

SECONDARY CENTRES OF OSSIFICATION

These appear at puberty and fuse in the third decade

AT PUBERTY

Annular ossification includes facets for ribs

Neurocentral fusion

Centres for transverse process and spine

Annular ossification in epiphyseal plate

The skull

Initially, the developing brain is supported by a *plate of mesenchyme*. The plate encases the cranial end of the notochord and extends anteriorly and laterally to become continuous with the *mesenchymatous capsules* of the sense organs. Beyond and between them the plate is continuous with the *general head mesenchyme* surrounding the brain. Ventrally the plate is continuous with the *mesenchyme of the pharyngeal arches*. Centres of *chondrification* representing the components of the primitive skull appear and fuse to form a continuous *base* to the *neurocranium*. Sites of fusion are indicated by foramina through which the cranial nerves leave the skull. From a *parachordal centre*, chondrification extends through the unsegmented paraxial mesoderm anterior to the somite region, through the fused sclerotomes of the occipital region (where it encloses the roots of the hypoglossal nerve) and around the neural tube (where it bounds the foramen magnum). The resulting occipital cartilage forms most of the future occipital bone. Occipital cartilage fuses with the medial and posterior aspects of the otic capsule, which is now chondrified, and entraps the glossopharyngeal, vagus and accessory nerves in the jugular foramen. The otic capsule (future petromastoid temporal bone) is defective medially where the facial and vestibulocochlear nerves enter the internal acoustic meatus. From *polar and trabecular centres*, flanking the developing hypophysis and between it and the nasal capsules, chondrification extends through mesenchyme derived (experiments suggest) from the prechordal plate and, anteriorly, from the neural crest. The polar centres form postsphenoid cartilage which extends around the hypophysis and backwards to fuse with parachordal cartilage. Trabecular chondrification forms presphenoid cartilage which extends forwards to fuse with cartilage which has developed around the olfactory pits and which gives rise to the ethmoid bone, the inferior conchae and the cartilaginous nasal septum. On either side of the polar and trabecular regions, chondrification *centres for the wings of the sphenoid* appear. The centre for the lesser wing sends medial extensions around the optic nerve to fuse with presphenoid cartilage and form the optic foramen. Posterior to this centre and separating it from the centre for the root of the greater wing are the oculomotor, trochlear, ophthalmic, maxillary and abducent nerves. The maxillary nerve is later encircled by cartilage, which grows anteriorly from the centre for the root of the greater wing, so that it is isolated in the foramen rotundum from the other nerves in the superior orbital fissure. The same cartilage extends posteriorly around the mandibular nerve to form the foramen ovale, and medially to fuse with postsphenoid cartilage. From the latter a bar extends back to the otic capsule and encloses the internal carotid artery in the carotid canal. Centres of *ossification* appear in the cartilaginous neurocranium and form the bones of the base of the skull.

The *roof* of the neurocranium does not chondrify, and the frontal, parietal and interparietal occipital bones ossify in *membrane*. The membrane bones which develop in apposition to the nasal capsule (e.g. nasal and lacrimal) and to the sides of the cartilaginous neurocranium (e.g. squamous temporal and most of the greater wing of the sphenoid) clearly have some claim to be considered as derivatives of the neurocranium. However, because of morphological, developmental and functional affinities, they will be considered here as derivatives of the membranous viscerocranium.

Experiments indicate that the *viscerocranium* is almost completely developed in mesenchyme of neural crest origin. This mesenchyme contributes to the frontonasal prominence and to the pharyngeal arches, where it forms the *arch cartilages*.

Other parts of the viscerocranium ossify in *membrane* in the mixed mesenchyme of the facial prominences, often in apposition to cartilage. In the frontonasal prominence, centres appear for the nasal and lacrimal bones; whether or not there are premaxillary centres is disputed. On the deep aspect of the maxillary prominence, centres appear for the maxilla and the palatine bone and spread into the palatal process. A centre for the vomer appears in the maxillary mesenchyme of the nasal septum. In the depths of the maxillary prominence a centre for most of the greater wing of the sphenoid appears and spreads down into the pterygoid region. More superficially, centres appear for the zygomatic and squamous temporal bones. In the mandibular prominence a centre for the mandible appears lateral to Meckel's cartilage and a centre for the tympanic part of the temporal bone appears in relation to the external acoustic meatus.

GENERAL PLAN OF THE PRIMITIVE HUMAN SKULL

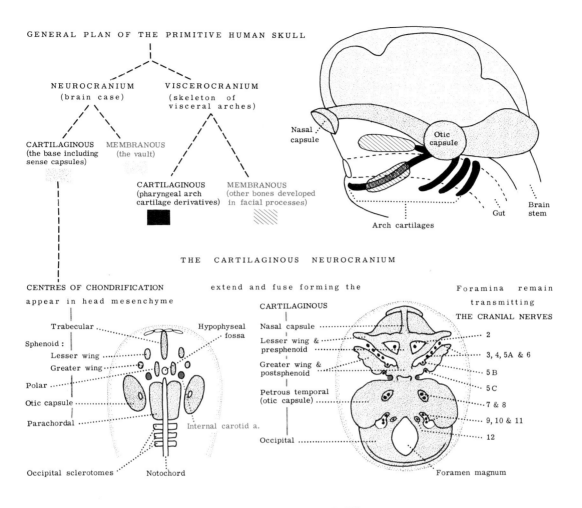

NEUROCRANIUM (brain case)

VISCEROCRANIUM (skeleton of visceral arches)

CARTILAGINOUS (the base including sense capsules)

MEMBRANOUS (the vault)

CARTILAGINOUS (pharyngeal arch cartilage derivatives)

MEMBRANOUS (other bones developed in facial processes)

Nasal capsule

Otic capsule

Gut

Brain stem

Arch cartilages

THE CARTILAGINOUS NEUROCRANIUM

CENTRES OF CHONDRIFICATION appear in head mesenchyme

Trabecular

Sphenoid :
Lesser wing
Greater wing

Polar

Otic capsule

Parachordal

Hypophyseal fossa

Internal carotid a.

Occipital sclerotomes

Notochord

extend and fuse forming the

CARTILAGINOUS

Nasal capsule

Lesser wing & presphenoid

Greater wing & postsphenoid

Petrous temporal (otic capsule)

Occipital

Foramina remain transmitting
THE CRANIAL NERVES

2

3, 4, 5A & 6

5 B

5 C

7 & 8

9, 10 & 11

12

Foramen magnum

DEFINITIVE DERIVATIVES

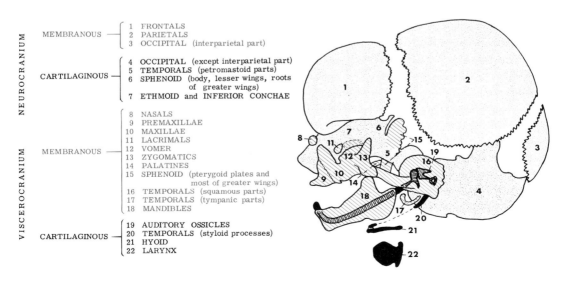

NEUROCRANIUM

MEMBRANOUS
1 FRONTALS
2 PARIETALS
3 OCCIPITAL (interparietal part)

CARTILAGINOUS
4 OCCIPITAL (except interparietal part)
5 TEMPORALS (petromastoid parts)
6 SPHENOID (body, lesser wings, roots of greater wings)
7 ETHMOID and INFERIOR CONCHAE

VISCEROCRANIUM

MEMBRANOUS
8 NASALS
9 PREMAXILLAE
10 MAXILLAE
11 LACRIMALS
12 VOMER
13 ZYGOMATICS
14 PALATINES
15 SPHENOID (pterygoid plates and most of greater wings)
16 TEMPORALS (squamous parts)
17 TEMPORALS (tympanic parts)
18 MANDIBLES

CARTILAGINOUS
19 AUDITORY OSSICLES
20 TEMPORALS (styloid processes)
21 HYOID
22 LARYNX

Bone and joints

Essentially, *ossification* is the mineralization of connective tissue. At the outset, mesenchyme condenses and its cells form rounded, metabolically active *osteoblasts* which make contact by thin processes in a semifluid ground substance. The osteoblasts secrete a structureless matrix around themselves and collagen fibrils are precipitated in it. The collagen fibrils mature and aggregate, and minute crystals of hydroxyapatite appear on, in and between them. As the crystals grow, they obscure the fibrillar pattern of the matrix. The cells and their processes become encased in bone as they become less metabolically active and form *osteocytes*. Meanwhile, further osteoblasts are recruited from the cells of the surrounding richly vascular tissue and form an osteogenic layer which repeats the process at the surface of the developing bony trabeculae. The mesenchyme persisting between the trabeculae gives rise to the endosteum and myeloid tissue of spongy bone, and the limiting membrane becomes the periosteum.

Bone-eroding multinucleated giant cells—*osteoclasts*—are probably derived from phagocytes which arrive via the bloodstream. As the bone grows, there is continual internal reconstruction. This entails a delicate balance between the depositional activity of osteoblasts and the resorptive activity of osteoclasts. Adequate blood levels of calcium and phosphate and incompletely determined but critical local cellular factors (e.g. *matrix vesicles*) are necessary for normal bone formation.

The *membranous neurocranium* consists of a single continuous layer of condensed mesenchyme. Individual centres of ossification appear in the membrane and spread centrifugally, splitting the mesenchyme into two *limiting membranes*. The external membrane forms the periosteum and the internal membrane forms the dura mater. Each has a *fibrous layer* and an *osteogenic layer* containing osteoblasts. These layers are continuous around and between the advancing edges of the bones. The advancing edges meet at *sutures* (bone–fibrous tissue–bone) where active growth continues. Within the *facial prominences*, centres of ossification are surrounded only by an *osteogenic layer* and spread through looser mesenchyme. Limiting fibrous layers are formed only when the bones meet at sutures. In the vault and the facial skeleton, sutures are active growth mechanisms during fetal life and childhood due to the depositional activity of the osteoblasts. At varying times growth at

sutures becomes quiescent as the *interzone* thins, and most sutures eventually ossify.

In other situations several stages precede what is essentially the same process of *ossification*. Fibrils appear in the intercellular substance of the condensed mesenchyme of the blastemal skeleton. They are then obscured by the basophil secretions of cells which have enlarged and become rounded *chondroblasts*. Thus are formed rather precise cartilaginous models of future bones, each surrounded by a limiting membrane. Ossification then occurs directly beneath the limiting membrane and forms a *periosteal bone collar* around the cartilaginous model. Within the last, phases of swelling, degeneration, provisional calcification and erosion by vascular mesenchyme precede ossification proper. After a primitive marrow cavity is formed by erosion, *endosteal bone* is deposited on remnants of calcified cartilage and on the inner aspect of the periosteal collar. The process of ossification and internal and external reconstruction extends along the length of the bone towards the epiphyses, where growth of cartilage continues.

Long before birth, *cartilage canals* containing vascular mesenchyme pervade the epiphyses and supply them with nutrients. Much later, usually after birth, ossification spreads from a centrally eroded cavity in the epiphysis until only a rim of growth cartilage remains. An *epiphyseal plate* of growth cartilage remains to separate epiphyseal from metaphyseal bone and a so-called *primary cartilaginous joint* (bone–hyaline cartilage–bone) is formed.

At first, the epiphyseal plate is active on both surfaces as its cells proliferate and lay down cartilage to be replaced by epiphyseal and metaphyseal bone. The distal (epiphyseal) surface of the growth cartilage then becomes quiescent and an epiphyseal bone plate is separated from the zone of proliferation by a zone of resting cells, one or two cells thick. Thereafter, growth in length is achieved mainly by the replacement of cartilage laid down on the proximal (metaphyseal) aspect of the growth cartilage. Growth continues until this process ceases, the cartilage then being completely replaced by bone. Similar temporary joints permit skull and vertebral growth.

Centrifugal growth in a flat bone is accompanied by changes of curvature. Longitudinal growth in a long bone is accompanied by changes in diameter, particularly at the ends where the metaphysis of one stage is incorporated into the diaphysis of the next. These changes are produced by balanced activity of periosteal and endosteal bone deposition and resorption.

Intramembranous Ossification

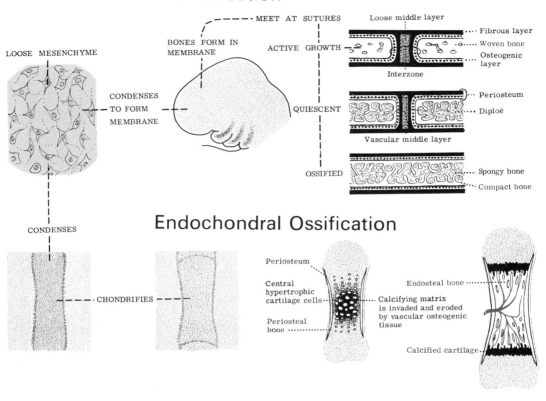

LOOSE MESENCHYME

CONDENSES TO FORM MEMBRANE

MEET AT SUTURES

BONES FORM IN MEMBRANE

ACTIVE GROWTH

Loose middle layer

Fibrous layer
Woven bone
Osteogenic layer

Interzone

QUIESCENT

Periosteum
Diploë

Vascular middle layer

OSSIFIED

Spongy bone
Compact bone

CONDENSES

Endochondral Ossification

CHONDRIFIES

Periosteum

Central hypertrophic cartilage cells

Periosteal bone

Calcifying matrix is invaded and eroded by vascular osteogenic tissue

Calcified cartilage

Endosteal bone

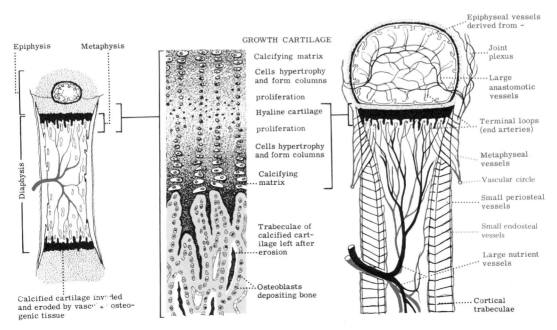

Epiphysis   Metaphysis

Diaphysis

GROWTH CARTILAGE

Calcifying matrix

Cells hypertrophy and form columns

proliferation

Hyaline cartilage

proliferation

Cells hypertrophy and form columns

Calcifying matrix

Trabeculae of calcified cartilage left after erosion

Osteoblasts depositing bone

Calcified cartilage invaded and eroded by vascular osteogenic tissue

Epiphyseal vessels derived from –

Joint plexus

Large anastomotic vessels

Terminal loops (end arteries)

Metaphyseal vessels

Vascular circle

Small periosteal vessels

Small endosteal vessels

Large nutrient vessels

Cortical trabeculae

Fetal bone is classified as *woven bone*, since its collagenous fibres vary in size and interweave irregularly. Only postnatally does bone become compacted and organized. Thus, at birth, the flat bones of the skull consist of single plates of woven bone, and the shafts of long bones are also largely made up of this type. After birth, woven bone is compacted by the deposition of *lamellar bone* on its trabeculae, filling up the interstices. Similar finely and regularly fibred lamellar bone is deposited beneath the periosteum and endosteum. The internal architecture of this early bone depends largely upon the vascular pattern within it. Concentric deposition of lamellae within primary vascular spaces produces *Haversian systems* or *primary osteons*. As bone develops, *secondary osteons* are formed by the deposition of lamellae within canals resulting from the resorption of pre-existing bone and become the structural units of compact or cortical bone.

Spongy bone consists of a meshwork of trabeculae in which lamellar organization is less regular. Only a few large trabeculae contain blood vessels. The others are sustained by surrounding vessels. By means of balanced deposition and resorption, the trabeculae become organized in response to stress (Wolff's law). Many trabeculae are orientated along lines of stress. Others intersect them and act as struts or tie beams. Alterations in stress pattern lead to alterations in trabecular pattern.

The suture and so-called primary cartilaginous joint are temporary structures and are essentially growth mechanisms which permit little or no movement between the skeletal units they connect. *Secondary cartilaginous joints* (bone–hyaline cartilage–fibrocartilage–hyaline cartilage–bone) are usually permanent structures which permit limited movement. They are found only in the midline of the body where cartilaginous models of bones meet. Each cartilaginous model is surrounded by a limiting membrane—the *perichondrium*—which has an outer *fibrous layer* and an inner *chondrogenic layer* containing chondroblasts. These layers are continuous around and between the ends of the models as they approach each other within the blastemal skeleton. When they meet, three layers may be distinguished within the interzone of condensed mesenchyme trapped between them. The chondrogenic layers at the ends of the models are the sites of appositional growth. Between them is a single intermediate layer which represents the fibrous layers of the perichondria. Cartilage is not the primary tissue in the intermediate layer, but cartilage cells appear later, as a secondary phenomenon, and transform the fibrous tissue into fibrocartilage. Meanwhile, ossification spreads through the cartilage and nears the joint. A layer of hyaline growth cartilage caps the bone and persists for a while as active growth continues. Later, growth becomes quiescent and the cap is reduced to a thin plate flanking the fibrocartilage. This last may develop a non-synovial cleft. Such joints do not usually ossify.

Synovial joints (bone–cartilage–synovial cavity–cartilage–bone) are permanent and permit more or less free movement. As elsewhere, the blastemal skeleton of condensed mesenchyme is continuous across the site of the future joint. Again, as the cartilaginous models grow towards each other, condensed mesenchyme forms an interzone between them. At first this interzone is homogeneous but soon it shows the same three layers as that of the secondary cartilaginous joint. The peripheral part of the intermediate layer—*blastemal synovial mesenchyme*—lies beneath a primitive joint capsule derived from the limiting membrane of the blastemal skeleton. Blood vessels then grow into the perichondria and the capsular area but not into the chondrogenic layers or the more central intermediate layer of the interzone. The primordia of intra-articular soft tissues, such as fat pads, folds and synovial tissue generally, become recognizable in the vascularized synovial mesenchyme. As the tissue of the intermediate layer loosens, the primordia of intra-articular structures, such as ligaments and menisci, become apparent within it. Collagen fibres begin to appear in these structures, in the joint capsule, and in the extra-articular ligaments which differentiate from it. The cells of the intermediate layer surround themselves with cartilaginous matrix and are incorporated into the subjacent layers, which cease to be chondrogenic. In this way the intermediate layer thins and disappears, leaving a central joint cavity which spreads peripherally. Small joint surfaces may appear to fuse at this stage (e.g. in the carpus and tarsus) but this may be artefactual. It does not occur in larger joints, where it would certainly be prevented by movement. The joint cavity spreads throughout the area previously occupied by the avascular intermediate zone until vascular synovial mesenchyme is reached and its derivatives are outlined.

The cells from which the skeleton is formed are determined very early in development and the blastemal skeleton is self-differentiating (p. 114).

Symphyses

DEVELOPING

Fibrous layer

Chondrogenic layer

Cartilage

Interzone

Perichondrium

ACTIVE GROWTH

Osteogenic layer

Cap of growth cartilage

Woven bone

Fibrocartilage

Periosteum

QUIESCENT

Spongy bone

Compact bone

Cleft

Synovial Joints

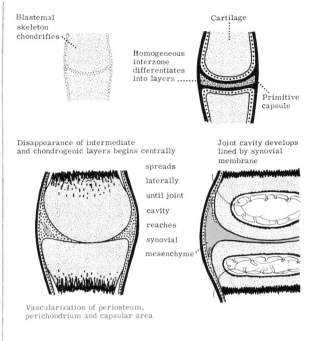

Blastemal skeleton chondrifies

Cartilage

Homogeneous interzone differentiates into layers

Primitive capsule

Disappearance of intermediate and chondrogenic layers begins centrally

spreads

laterally

until joint

cavity

reaches

synovial

mesenchyme

Joint cavity develops lined by synovial membrane

Vascularization of periosteum, perichondrium and capsular area

ADULT

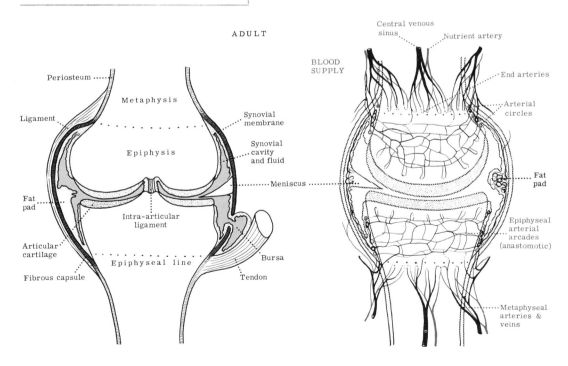

Periosteum

Metaphysis

Ligament

Synovial membrane

Epiphysis

Synovial cavity and fluid

Meniscus

Fat pad

Intra-articular ligament

Articular cartilage

Epiphyseal line

Bursa

Fibrous capsule

Tendon

BLOOD SUPPLY

Central venous sinus

Nutrient artery

End arteries

Arterial circles

Fat pad

Epiphyseal arterial arcades (anastomotic)

Metaphyseal arteries & veins

111

The limbs

Limb buds are first seen towards the end of the somite stage as slight longitudinal ridges on the body wall (somatopleure) immediately ventral to the lower cervical and upper sacral somites (p. 64). Limb mesoderm is determined very early and its proliferation induces a thickening (*ridge*) in the overlying (*apical*) ectoderm. As the buds grow they become rounded, and then rather flattened dorsoventrally. They soon show a distinct internal organization. A capillary plexus develops in the mesenchyme of the bud, taps the intersegmental arteries which are differentiating in its base, and drains into a *marginal vein*. The apical ridge of ectoderm overlies the vein. It appears that the apical ridge and the marginal vein are both essential to the activity of *apical mesoderm*, which lays down the segments of the limb in proximodistal order.

At this stage the flexor aspect of the limb is ventral, the extensor aspect is dorsal, and the preaxial and postaxial borders are cranial and caudal respectively. The cells of the dermatomes and the related spinal nerves are distributed in segmental bands around the trunk and on the limb bud. The fifth cervical nerve supplies a preaxial strip of arm bud, the first thoracic a postaxial strip, and intermediate nerves parallel strips between them. The nerves supply both dorsal and ventral surfaces. The growing limb bud develops a paddle-shaped end, the smooth outline of which is soon broken by the active growth of five digital rudiments and necrosis of the tissues around and between them. As the limb elongates, the distribution of the intermediate nerves migrates along it so that they no longer reach the surface of the proximal part. Dorsal and ventral *axial lines* may then be defined. These lines separate adjacent areas of skin which are supplied by non-adjacent segments of the spinal cord (e.g. C4/T2). Adjacent segments overlap in their cutaneous distribution, but overlap across the lines is minimal. *A segmental nerve deficit, unrevealed by testing segmental skin areas consecutively, may be revealed by testing across the axial lines.*

Meanwhile *flexion creases* indicating the sites of future joints have appeared and the flexor aspect of each limb faces medially. By the beginning of the fetal period both limbs have rotated about their long axes, but in opposite directions, so that in the conventional anatomical position the flexor aspect of the arm faces anteriorly, and that of the leg, posteriorly. The preaxial nerves are now distributed to the lateral side of the arm and the anteromedial aspect of the leg, while the axial lines have undergone some distortion. Nevertheless, the sequence of segmental representation may still be traced along the preaxial side of the axial line and back along the postaxial side. Distally, the skin of the limbs shows specialization. Epidermal thickenings, representing the foot pads of lower mammals, make a transitory appearance, and nails and friction ridges develop. The pattern of the latter (fingerprints) is established early in the fetal period and persists throughout life.

At first, the capillary plexus of each limb bud is connected with several intersegmental arteries but soon the main *axial artery* differentiates from the plexus in continuity with branches of the seventh cervical or fifth lumbar artery, and other connections are lost. Each axial artery lies between flexor and extensor premuscle masses and ends in a capillary plexus which supplies the distal segment of the limb. In the *upper limb bud* the axial artery forms the axillary, brachial and anterior interosseous arteries. The posterior interosseous and median arteries differentiate as collateral branches. For a time the median artery feeds the distal capillary plexus, but when the radial and ulnar arteries appear they take over this function. The marginal vein forms the cephalic vein (preaxial), the basilic vein (postaxial) and the dorsal venous arch. In the *lower limb bud* the axial artery is soon largely superseded and persists only as the inferior gluteal artery, the artery to the sciatic nerve, and parts of the popliteal and peroneal arteries. With the medial rotation of the lower limb, the femoral and profunda femoris arteries differentiate and the axial artery is bypassed as the femoral artery joins it above the knee. Below the knee, collaterals develop and form the anterior and posterior tibial and proximal part of the peroneal arteries. The marginal vein forms the great saphenous vein (preaxial), the small saphenous vein (postaxial) and the dorsal venous arch. As blood vessels develop by haemodynamic selection within a vascular network, it is not surprising that anomalies are common. The great saphenous vein may enter the femoral vein at a lower level than usual. The latter may then be ligated in error at operation for varicose veins. The forearm arteries may originate high in the arm and lie superficially in the cubital fossa. They may then receive injections intended for the median cubital vein, with disastrous consequences.

Segmental Cutaneous Innervation

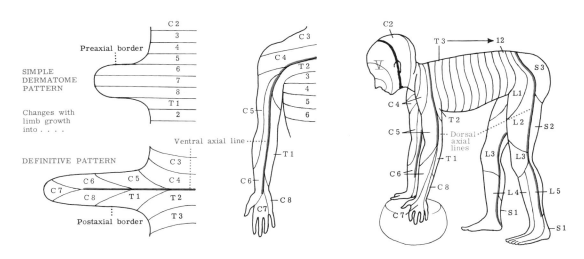

SIMPLE
DERMATOME
PATTERN

Changes with
limb growth
into . . . .

DEFINITIVE PATTERN

Preaxial border

C 2
3
4
5
6
7
8
T 1
2

Ventral axial line

C 3
C 4
C 5
C 6
C 7
C 8
T 1
T 2
T 3

Postaxial border

C 3
T 2
3
4
5
6
C 5
T 1
C 6
C 7
C 8

C2
T 3 → 12
S 3
C 4
L1
T 2
L 2
S 2
C 5
Dorsal axial lines
L3
L3
C 6
T 1
L 4
L 5
C 8
S 1
C 7
S 1

The Limb Arteries

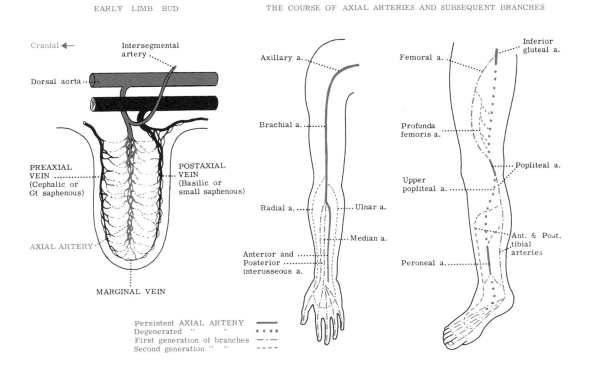

EARLY LIMB BUD

THE COURSE OF AXIAL ARTERIES AND SUBSEQUENT BRANCHES

Cranial ←

Intersegmental artery

Dorsal aorta

PREAXIAL VEIN
(Cephalic or Gt saphenous)

POSTAXIAL VEIN
(Basilic or small saphenous)

AXIAL ARTERY

MARGINAL VEIN

Axillary a.

Brachial a.

Radial a.

Ulnar a.

Median a.

Anterior and Posterior interosseous a.

Femoral a.

Inferior gluteal a.

Profunda femoris a.

Popliteal a.

Upper popliteal a.

Ant. & Post. tibial arteries

Peroneal a.

Persistent AXIAL ARTERY ——
Degenerated   "   "   • • • •
First generation of branches —·—·
Second generation "   "   —— ——

113

Limb mesenchyme is self-differentiating. Within it, *type* (forelimb or hindlimb), *polarity* (flexor aspect—anterior or posterior) and *internal structure* are determined and are independent of somites or of level of nerve supply. While blood vessels have been developing in loose mesenchyme, adjacent mesenchyme cells have proliferated and compacted, forming the blastemal limb skeleton. This is a single mass of condensed mesenchyme continuous across the sites of future joints. Within it centres of chondrification for individual bones appear. Cells round up and secrete a basophil intercellular substance which obscures the collagenous fibrils between them. From these centres, chondrification spreads within the blastemal skeleton until cartilaginous models of the bones, enclosed by perichondria and separated by mesenchymal interzones, are complete. By the beginning of the fetal period, these models have increased in size and fined down in proportion until they closely resemble the future bone. Given a suitable natural environment or culture medium, the general form of bones and joints, chondrification and early ossification all depend on intrinsic factors alone. Later, extrinsic factors, such as mechanical forces, also play their part. If a presumptive joint region is excised from the blastemal skeleton the remaining tissue is redistributed and joint formation is not prevented. A similar experiment after chondrification has begun results in fusion and lack of a joint.

Muscles are first indicated as premuscle masses of condensed mesenchyme in the base of the limb bud. *Myoblasts* become spindle-shaped and arranged in parallel bundles in which they fuse end to end, forming long multinucleate *myotubes*. Myofibrils appear within the myotubes and, increasing in number and size, develop cross-striations. The final number of fibres in a muscle is reached some time before birth. Muscles then grow by the increase in length and thickness of individual fibres and by the addition of myoblasts at their ends. As differentiation proceeds proximodistally within the limb bud, premuscle masses are formed dorsal and ventral to the developing bone. *Flexor and adductor muscles* develop in the *ventral mass* and *extensor and abductor muscles* in the *dorsal mass*. Some muscles, such as the latissimus dorsi, migrate and gain secondary attachments to the axial skeleton. The pectoral muscles and sternum are primarily appendicular, being derived from lateral plate mesoderm. Bilateral sternal plates of condensed mesenchyme appear ventral to, and independent of, costal processes as they advance through the body wall. The plates chondrify, fusing with each other and, secondarily, with the costal cartilages.

The *segmental spinal nerve* which grows out from the neural tube towards each myotome contains an admixture of motor and sensory fibres. The myotome and the spinal nerve divide into dorsal and ventral parts. The dorsal parts of the myotomes form the extensor muscles of the back. The *dorsal (posterior primary) rami* of the spinal nerves are mixed nerves supplying these muscles and the overlying skin segmentally. The ventral parts of the myotomes form the prevertebral muscles and the muscles of the body wall. The *ventral (anterior primary) rami* are mixed nerves supplying these muscles and the overlying skin segmentally. Certain of them (C5–T1 and L2–S3) also supply the muscles and skin of the limbs.

As the muscles of the limbs are laid down in proximodistal sequence, ventral rami reach them in craniocaudal sequence, so that the fifth cervical and second lumbar nerves are distributed to the proximal muscles, and the first thoracic and third sacral to the distal muscles. Each *ventral ramus* divides into *anterior* and *posterior divisions* which supply the *flexors* and *extensors* respectively. The picture is complicated by the formation of *plexuses*. Here, fibres which have been grouped by origin as segmental nerves become regrouped for distribution as *peripheral nerves*. Each segmental nerve is distributed to several peripheral nerves. Most peripheral nerves receive fibres from several segmental nerves.

That fibres from diverse origins should regroup as a peripheral nerve is not surprising since the direction of an outgrowing nerve fibre depends in part upon the ultrastructural orientation of the colloidal intercellular matrix through which it moves. Growth and migration produce alterations of orientation in the matrix and are followed by the earliest pioneer fibres. Subsequent fibres depend also upon contact guidance by the pioneer fibres and supporting cells. In the case of *axial musculature*, the migration and fusion of myotomes is a potent reason for the convergence of fibres from several segmental nerves on a single muscle. *Appendicular musculature* develops in situ in somatopleuric mesenchyme but shows a similar pattern of innervation. This is a reflection of the multisegmental origin of limb muscles in phylogeny. In man, muscles concerned with precise movements may be innervated from a single spinal segment. Without innervation, muscles may differentiate but they soon undergo fatty degeneration and are eventually absorbed. Although innervation from any level will prevent this, innervation from cervical or lumbar segments is necessary for normal co-ordinated limb function.

Early Forelimb Skeleton

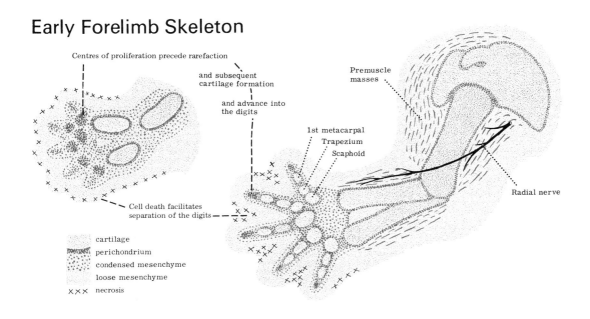

Centres of proliferation precede rarefaction

and subsequent cartilage formation

and advance into the digits

1st metacarpal
Trapezium
Scaphoid

Premuscle masses

Radial nerve

Cell death facilitates separation of the digits

cartilage
perichondrium
condensed mesenchyme
loose mesenchyme
××× necrosis

Plexuses and Muscle Innervation

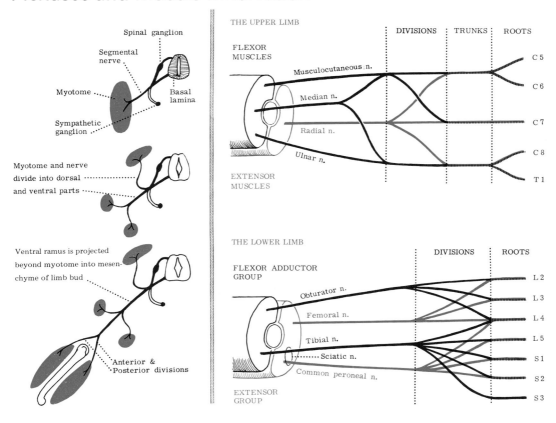

Spinal ganglion
Segmental nerve
Myotome
Sympathetic ganglion
Basal lamina

Myotome and nerve divide into dorsal and ventral parts

Ventral ramus is projected beyond myotome into mesenchyme of limb bud

Anterior & Posterior divisions

THE UPPER LIMB

DIVISIONS TRUNKS ROOTS

FLEXOR MUSCLES

Musculocutaneous n.   C 5
                           C 6
Median n.
Radial n.   C 7
Ulnar n.   C 8
EXTENSOR MUSCLES   T 1

THE LOWER LIMB

DIVISIONS ROOTS

FLEXOR ADDUCTOR GROUP

Obturator n.   L 2
                           L 3
Femoral n.   L 4
Tibial n.   L 5
Sciatic n.   S 1
Common peroneal n.   S 2
EXTENSOR GROUP   S 3

Anomalies

Amongst the commonest congenital anomalies are three involving the locomotor system—spina bifida, club foot and congenital dislocation of the hip.

In all cases of *spina bifida* there is non-union of one or more paired vertebral arches and, as a result, a cleft spine. However, the non-union may be primary—*spina bifida occulta*—or be secondary to a failure in the formation of the neural tube or the meninges—*spina bifida cystica* (p. 142). There is a craniocaudal gradient of union of paired vertebral arches and thus a differential incidence in the sites at which spina bifida occulta is found. Non-union caudally results in the normal sacral hiatus, most commonly between the laminae of the fourth and fifth parts of the sacrum but frequently extending higher; in nearly 3 per cent of all individuals a bony posterior wall to the sacral canal is completely lacking. Non-union of the first sacral vertebral arch is very common (1 in 8) and that of the fifth lumbar rather less (1 in 40); higher lesions are correspondingly less common. Spina bifida occulta is usually an incidental finding at radiological examination. However, if one or more vertebral spines and hence attachments of the erector spinae muscle are absent, it may be associated with flattening of the overlying contours and with low back pain. The presence of an adventitious tuft of hair may be the clue to the involvement of deeper structures.

Variations in the number of coccygeal segments are common but nearly all columns have 24 presacral vertebrae. However, due to *sacralization of the fifth lumbar* (cranial variation), some have only 23 presacral vertebrae whereas others, due to *lumbarization of the first sacral* segment (caudal variation), have 25. Cranial variation may include cervical ribs associated with the seventh cervical vertebra. A *cervical rib* may be complete, and articulate with the manubrium, or incomplete, in which case it may be represented wholly or in its anterior part by a fibrous band; it may produce compression of the neurovascular bundle entering the upper limb. *Spondylolisthesis*—forward displacement of a vertebral body on the one below—is not congenital nor has it a congenital basis.

Defects of the vault of skull, like those of the vertebral arches, may be primary or secondary to anomalies of neural tube formation or of the meninges (p. 142). Small defects without underlying anomalies may be palpable or evident only on radiological examination. In the rare *craniofacial synostoses*, some of which are familial, premature closure of one or more sutures results in anomalies of skull shape; some have proved amenable to surgery. In *microcephaly* the failure of the skull to expand is secondary to failure of the brain to grow and there is mental retardation.

Achondroplasia is a disturbance of growth and ossification in cartilage which, however, spares the vertebrae: the short skull base results in a saddle nose and often a minor degree of hydrocephalus and thus a bulging forehead; the short limb bones result in *dwarfism*. In its classic form, achondroplasia is an autosomal dominant trait.

Craniocleidal dysostosis is a disturbance of ossification in membrane and is also an autosomal dominant trait. The bones of the vault of the skull are separated by wide sutures and fontanelles; the face is small; the clavicles are deficient or absent, and so the shoulders can be brought together in front of the chest.

Normal development of the limbs requires not only the basic tissues and mechanisms but also fetal movements. If movements are impaired early, joints develop imperfectly; if they are confined later, the *congenital postural deformities* (p. 168) of club foot and congenital dislocation of the hip may result; both are multifactorial traits. In *club foot (talipes equinovarus)*, which is commoner in males, the sole of the foot is turned inwards and the foot is adducted and plantarflexed. *Congenital dislocation of the hip* is commoner in females and in breech presentations; the associated deficiency of the acetabular rim is a polygenic trait, and abnormal joint laxity, which may also contribute, is a monogenic trait.

Since the mesodermal components of a limb are laid down in proximodistal sequence, disturbance of the apical ectoderm/marginal vein complex at successively later times may result in absence of the limb—*amelia*; in absence or defect of its distal half—*hemimelia*; or in absence or defect of the hands or feet or digits. Secondary interference with a normally laid down limb may, in addition, result in interference with the intermediate part of the limb so that the hand or foot is attached more or less directly to the trunk—*phocomelia (seal flipper; meromelia)*. Most reduction deformities of the limbs have a hereditary basis, although in the early 1960s many resulted from pregnant women taking the drug thalidomide (p. 26). Among other effects, this drug damages the axial artery of the limb bud and most commonly produces phocomelia.

Polydactyly, in which there are supernumerary digits, may result from an abnormal zone of proliferative activity at the periphery of the limb bud. *Syndactyly*, in which the digits are more or less fused, may result from failure of the normal mechanism of their separation by cell death. In *lobster claw hand* the third digit is missing and an abnormal cleft extending into the palm separates the fused first/second and fourth/fifth digits. In the very rare condition *sympodia* the lower limbs are fused and may be reduced to a tapering remnant. Significantly, if the knees are developed they face backwards, the soles forwards and the great toes are on the outside—i.e. the normal medial rotation of the lower limbs has not occurred.

SPINA BIFIDA OCCULTA

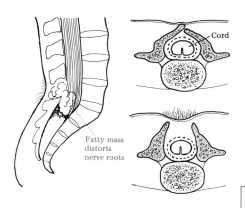

Cord

Fatty mass distorts nerve roots

VARIATIONS OF THE SACRUM

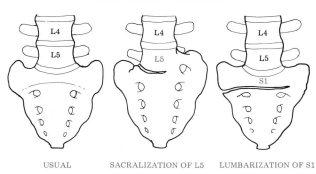

USUAL   SACRALIZATION OF L5   LUMBARIZATION OF S1

VARIETIES OF CERVICAL RIB

1 Unusually long transverse process

2 Minute cervical rib

3 Long cervical rib reaching to 1st rib or costal cartilage or may end freely

4 Complete cervical rib articulating with manubrium

5 Fibrous band connecting tip of transverse process or cervical rib to scalene tubercle

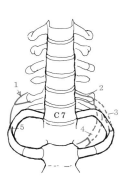

ACHONDROPLASTIC DWARFISM

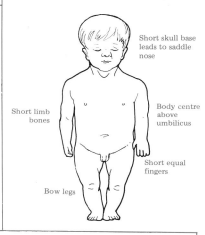

Short skull base leads to saddle nose

Short limb bones

Body centre above umbilicus

Short equal fingers

Bow legs

CLEIDOCRANIAL DYSOSTOSIS

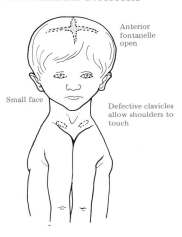

Anterior fontanelle open

Small face

Defective clavicles allow shoulders to touch

TALIPES EQUINOVARUS

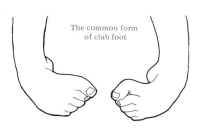

The common form of club foot

CONGENITAL DISLOCATION OF THE HIP

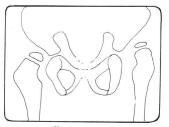

X-ray appearance

MICROCEPHALY

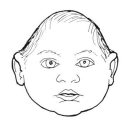

PHOCOMELIA

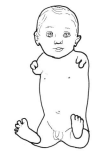

PREAXIAL POLYDACTYLY

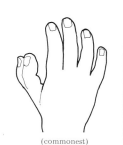

(commonest)

SYNDACTYLY

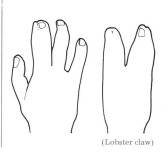

(Lobster claw)

SYMPODIA

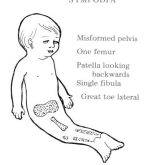

Misformed pelvis
One femur
Patella looking backwards
Single fibula
Great toe lateral

117

The Skin and Adnexa

The epidermis, hairs, nails, sebaceous and sweat glands are developed from general body ectoderm to which the neural crest contributes melanoblasts. The dermis is derived in part from the dermatomic cells of the somite and in part from somatopleuric mesenchyme of mixed lateral plate and neural crest origin.

The simple cuboidal ectoderm soon forms two layers: an outer, temporarily protective, layer of flat cells—the *epitrichium*; and the *primitive epidermis*. The layers of the *definitive epidermis* appear after repeated mitotic divisions and differentiation in the primitive layer. By mid-pregnancy the various stages of keratinization are present, and basal cell, prickle cell, granular, clear and horny layers may be distinguished. The epitrichium, too, is keratinized and begins to be shed. With cells of the horny layer and sebaceous secretions it forms the *vernix caseosa*—a cheesy material which in the latter half of pregnancy covers the fetal skin and helps to resist maceration by amniotic fluid.

Meanwhile, mesenchyme condenses and forms the dermis. Some of the cells form fibroblasts which lay down a feltwork of dermal collagen and elastic fibres. Others form the capillary and the lymphatic plexuses of the dermis and the cells of the subcutaneous areolar tissue. As term approaches, these become laden with fat, producing the rounded contours of the full-term child. The dermoepidermal junction is at first flat but soon develops corrugations—the dermal papillae—over which the epidermis becomes moulded.

The *hairs* develop from solid cylindrical downgrowths of the epidermis, which grow into the underlying mesenchyme. The tip of each downgrowth becomes bulbous and the margins of the bulb grow around a vascular mesodermal condensation— the hair papilla. The central cells of the epidermal downgrowth proliferate and elongate. They develop keratin within their cytoplasm and form the shaft of the hair. The peripheral cells of the epidermal downgrowth form the inner *root sheath* of the hair follicle. A series of flask-shaped outgrowths from this inner sheath form the sebaceous glands. The surrounding mesenchyme cells condense and form the outer root sheath of the hair follicle. Some of the cells differentiate into the smooth muscle strands of the arrector pili and connect secondarily with the root sheath. As proliferation continues, the apex of the hair approaches the surface layers, which it pierces. The first hairs to appear are extremely fine and are termed *lanugo*. This largely disappears in the later months of pregnancy. The definitive hairs occasionally arise from pre-existing lanugo follicles, but mainly from new generations of follicles.

The *sweat glands* develop as solid cylindrical downgrowths of ectoderm. The deeper part of the downgrowth coils on itself and forms the body of the gland. Later, the central cells degenerate and form a lumen which is surrounded by secretory cells in the body of the gland and by passive duct-lining cells in the uncoiled superficial parts. Around the secretory cells, ectodermal cells differentiate into contractile myoepitheliocytes.

The *nail* rudiment first appears as a thickened ectodermal plaque (*primary nail field*) at the tip of the digit. From there it migrates on to the dorsal aspect of the terminal phalanx but retains its innervation from the ventral aspect. With superficial keratinization, each primary nail field forms a false nail, whose margins are soon marked by deep proximal and shallow lateral nail folds. The true nail consists of modified clear layer, and grows, from the depths of the proximal nail fold, over the nail bed. At first the nail is covered superficially by a layer of eponychium derived from the false nail, but by term the edge of the nail has reached the tip of the digit and the eponychium has disappeared, except around the curved rim of the nail fold.

The *milk ridges* are linear ectodermal thickenings which extend over the ventral body wall, between the bases of the limb buds on each side. Normally the ridges are obvious only over the thorax where they form the breast primordia. The ectodermal thickening grows into the underlying mesenchyme, some 20 buds growing out from it. The buds branch and, nearer term, canalize to form the primitive secretory units, duct-lining cells and myoepitheliocytes. The fatty connective tissue of the breast develops from the surrounding mesenchyme. The nipple is at first a depressed zone which receives the orifices of the ducts. In the perinatal period it becomes everted by proliferation of the underlying mesenchyme. Growth of the male and female breasts is similar in childhood. At puberty, under the influence of oestrogens, the female breast hypertrophies and the areola develops and becomes lightly pigmented. Oestrogens primarily stimulate duct growth, whereas progesterone stimulates lobuloalveolar growth. During pregnancy both components hypertrophy and the nipple becomes further pigmented. The stimulus of prolactin is necessary for lactation, and suckling is necessary for its continuance. Supernumerary nipples or, rarely, breasts may develop at any point along the milk ridge.

The Skin and Hair

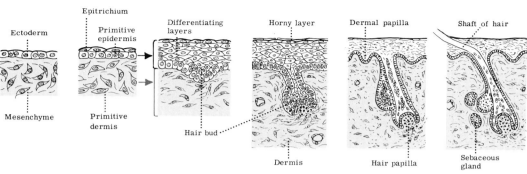

Ectoderm

Mesenchyme

Epitrichium

Primitive epidermis

Primitive dermis

Differentiating layers

Hair bud

Horny layer

Dermis

Dermal papilla

Hair papilla

Shaft of hair

Sebaceous gland

Sweat Gland

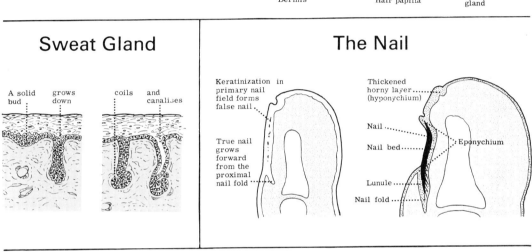

A solid bud

grows down

coils and canalises

The Nail

Keratinization in primary nail field forms false nail

True nail grows forward from the proximal nail fold

Thickened horny layer (hyponychium)

Nail

Nail bed

Lunule

Nail fold

Eponychium

The Breast

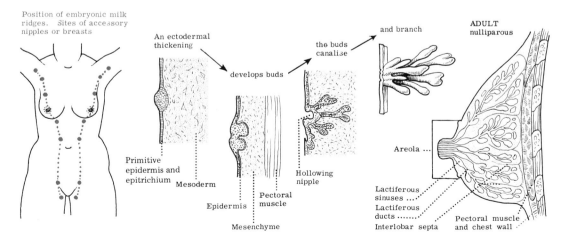

Position of embryonic milk ridges. Sites of accessory nipples or breasts

An ectodermal thickening

develops buds

the buds canalise

and branch

ADULT nulliparous

Primitive epidermis and epitrichium

Mesoderm

Epidermis

Mesenchyme

Pectoral muscle

Hollowing nipple

Areola

Lactiferous sinuses

Lactiferous ducts

Interlobar septa

Pectoral muscle and chest wall

119

The Teeth

As the jaws develop, the palate becomes separated from the upper lip, and the tongue from the lower lip, by a shallow *sulcus*. From the depths of each sulcus two *ectodermal laminae* arise. Like the sulcus, the laminae are U-shaped and follow the curves of the primitive jaws. The outer of the two epithelial laminae is termed *vestibular*, as its central cells break down to form the vestibule of the mouth. The inner of the two is the *dental lamina*. It soon develops ten centres of proliferation from which *buds* grow into the underlying mesenchyme. These are the primordia of the ectodermal part of the deciduous teeth. Each bud expands and forms an *epithelial dental (enamel) organ*. The cells on its deep aspect—the *inner dental epithelium*—become columnar and induce a vascular condensation in the mesenchyme which they cap—the *dental papilla*. The cells on the superficial aspect of the epithelial dental organ—the *outer dental epithelium*—remain cuboidal while the central cells of the organ form a *stellate reticulum*. The mesenchyme surrounding the dental organ and papilla forms a dense fibrous *dental sac.*

The inner dental epithelium is separated by a basement membrane from the peripheral cells of the dental papilla, and induces them to differentiate into columnar dentine-forming cells—the *odontoblasts*. The cell bodies of the odontoblasts move away from the basement membrane but remain connected with it by *dentinal processes*. Collagen fibres and an intercellular matrix are deposited around and between the processes to form *predentine*. Crystals of apatite are deposited around the fibres to form globular patches or layers which later fuse to give mature *dentine* a homogeneous appearance. The dentinal processes of the odontoblasts persist in *dentinal tubules* and their cell bodies remain at the surface of the dental papilla, which centrally becomes the *dental pulp*.

The cells of the stellate reticulum adjoining the inner dental epithelium flatten and form an *intermediate layer*. Both dentine and the intermediate layer are essential to *enamel* formation. The columnar cells of the inner dental epithelium become enamel-forming *ameloblasts*. The cell body of each ameloblast moves away from the basement membrane as its basal formative end secretes a granular proteinaceous matrix. The formative end continually adds to this preenamel matrix, which becomes progressively mineralized. Minute crystals of hydroxyapatite appear and the matrix becomes young enamel. Further crystallization, loss of water and reduction of the organic matrix forms mature enamel. The direction of crystal growth is primarily perpendicular to the formative end of the ameloblasts. The classical view that each produces a single oblique enamel rod with its base at the dentinoenamel junction is thus probably erroneous, the concept of rod and inter-rod enamel solely reflecting regional variations in crystal orientation. Meanwhile, the outer dental epithelium becomes corrugated as the mesenchyme of the dental sac forms vascular *papillae*. These supply the avascular dental organ with the nutrients necessary for its high metabolic activity, via the flattening stellate reticulum and the intermediate layer.

The dental lamina proliferates and gives rise to a bud which grows into the mesenchyme on the lingual aspect of each deciduous tooth germ. These buds form the epithelial dental organs of the *permanent teeth*, other than the molars. The dental organs of the permanent molars arise from an extension of the dental lamina beyond the second deciduous molar. The deciduous dentition is initiated in the postsomite embryo. The permanent teeth are initiated during the fetal period, in infancy and in childhood.

The part of the dental lamina which connects the epithelial dental organs with the oral epithelium is broken up by mesenchymal invasion, and disappears. At this stage the inner and outer dental epithelia meet at an acute angle beyond which they are in contact and proliferate to form the *root sheath*. Dentine and enamel formation begin at the apex of the dental papilla and spread towards the root sheath. Here the inner dental epithelium remains cuboidal. It does not produce enamel but does induce the formation of odontoblasts and, hence, of dentine.

Distally, new root sheath continues to form and to induce dentine formation until the apex of the root is established. Proximally, however, the mesenchyme of the dental sac breaks up the root sheath and comes into contact with the outer surface of the root dentine. The mesenchyme forms the *periodontal ligament* and its cells differentiate into three main types. The majority become fibroblasts which form the fibres of the ligament. The inner cells, adjoining the root dentine, become *cementoblasts* and deposit a layer of uncalcified cementoid substance, containing fibres, on the surface of the dentine. Cementoid becomes calcified to form cementum. The outer cells of the periodontal ligament become the periosteal osteoblasts of alveolar bone.

The form of the dentinoenamel and dentinocemental junctions is specific for each type of tooth and determines its definitive morphology. When enamel has completely developed and matured, the ameloblasts become flattened and indistinguishable from the intermediate layer and outer dental epithelium. Together they form a stratified covering—the *reduced enamel epithelium*—which produces an unmineralized cuticle over the enamel and protects it from resorption. The reduced enamel epithelium and oral epithelium over the crown of the tooth proliferate and fuse so that eruption occurs through an epithelial mass. Proliferating cells form the dentogingival *junctional epithelium* between enamel and oral epithelium.

The Teeth

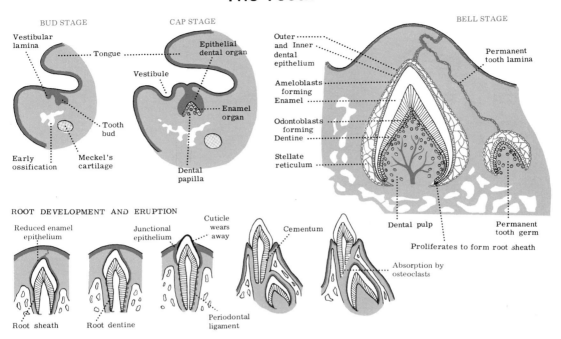

BUD STAGE

Vestibular lamina
Tongue
Tooth bud
Early ossification
Meckel's cartilage

CAP STAGE

Epithelial dental organ
Vestibule
Enamel organ
Dental papilla

BELL STAGE

Outer and Inner dental epithelium
Permanent tooth lamina
Ameloblasts forming Enamel
Odontoblasts forming Dentine
Stellate reticulum
Dental pulp
Permanent tooth germ
Proliferates to form root sheath

ROOT DEVELOPMENT AND ERUPTION

Reduced enamel epithelium
Junctional epithelium
Cuticle wears away
Cementum
Root sheath
Root dentine
Periodontal ligament
Absorption by osteoclasts

The Mandible

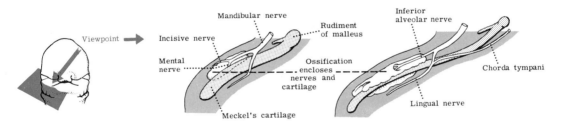

Viewpoint

Mandibular nerve
Incisive nerve
Mental nerve
Rudiment of malleus
Ossification encloses nerves and cartilage
Meckel's cartilage
Inferior alveolar nerve
Chorda tympani
Lingual nerve

SOME ASPECTS OF GROWTH

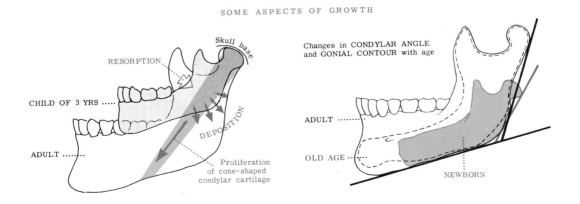

Skull base
RESORPTION
CHILD OF 3 YRS
DEPOSITION
ADULT
Proliferation of cone-shaped condylar cartilage

Changes in CONDYLAR ANGLE and GONIAL CONTOUR with age
ADULT
OLD AGE
NEWBORN

The Nervous System

Organization

The survival of an organism depends in part upon its capacity to react to its external environment, to respond to stimuli. In making a response, the relationship of the organism to the stimulus changes so that the events make up a closed loop—the *stimulus–response loop.*

In all but the simplest animals, nerve cells or *neurons* are specialized for the rapid conduction of information within the organism and form the pathways between cells which receive stimuli and cells which effect responses. *Sensory neurons* conduct electrical impulses, signals which convey information from the periphery, where they are generated at sensory endings or in sense organs, and deliver them into the central nervous system (CNS—spinal cord and brain). The signals which *motor neurons* receive from other neurons are combined (*integration*) into a total message which, if appropriate, is delivered to effector organs such as muscles and glands. The message may be modified (*modulation*) at the site of transfer of information from one neuron to another, a site which is called a *synapse.* In a monosynaptic reflex loop, information is transferred directly from a sensory neuron to a motor neuron. Usually, however, other neurons—*interneurons*—are interposed between the sensory and motor neurons so that the stimulus–response loop is polysynaptic and messages are subject to modulation and integration at additional sites, thus reducing the predictability of the response. Furthermore, while the activation of a monosynaptic loop is confined to one body segment, the inclusion of interneurons provides the basis for intersegmental and suprasegmental ('higher') influences on the activity of motor neurons.

Each neuron has processes, long or short, extending from a cell body which contains its nucleus. With few exceptions, the cell bodies of *sensory neurons* are located in the spinal and cranial nerve ganglia, and only their central processes enter the CNS (a *ganglion* is a collection of nerve cell bodies *outside* the CNS). The cell bodies of *somatic motor neurons* are located in the motor nuclei of the spinal cord and brain stem, and their peripheral processes leave the CNS to innervate striated muscle (a *nucleus* is a collection of nerve cell bodies *inside* the CNS). The cell bodies of *visceral motor neurons* are located in autonomic ganglia; they innervate smooth muscle, glands and fat. Thus sensory and motor neurons make up comparatively little of the CNS, the bulk of it being made up of vast numbers of cell bodies and processes of interneurons. The resulting myriads of synapses at which messages can be modified make possible the so-called higher functions, including memory, and further reduce the predictability of the response to a given stimulus.

Development

All neurons are derived from *ectoderm.* Under the influence of chorda-mesoderm, the ectoderm overlying it forms a thickened *neural plate* with a *neural ridge* at its periphery. The neural plate becomes grooved and the ridges on each side fold up into the amniotic cavity and meet in the midline to form the *neural tube.* At first the tube has open ends but these soon close. As the neural tube separates from the surface ectoderm, cells from the neural ridges form a *neural crest* in the angles between the tube and the surface.

Sensory and autonomic ganglia, and thus primary sensory and ganglionic visceral motor neurons, are derived from neural crest cells. *Sensory neuroblasts* (nerve-forming cells) send processes out to the periphery and into the neural tube which forms the CNS. *Visceral motor neuroblasts* send postganglionic processes out to innervate developing smooth muscle, glands and fat cells.

All other neurons (somatic motor neurons and interneurons) and their processes are derived from cells of the neural tube. *Somatic motor neuroblasts* send processes out of the CNS to innervate developing striated muscle. The neuroblasts of some interneurons (*visceral preganglionic neurons*) send processes out of the CNS to autonomic ganglia where they will form synapses with visceral motor neurons. The processes of neuroblasts of all other interneurons spread and make multitudinous synapses within the confines of the CNS.

The peripheral nervous system (spinal and cranial nerves, nerve roots, sensory and autonomic ganglia, plexuses and peripheral nerves) thus contains only sensory and visceral motor neurons plus the peripheral processes of somatic motor neurons and preganglionic visceral interneurons.

Even before the neural tube forms, the neural plate is expanded anteriorly in the region of the future brain. As the neural tube closes, this expanded part forms forebrain, midbrain and hindbrain vesicles while the unexpanded part forms the spinal cord. With further expansion and the formation of flexures, the brain becomes folded within the skull, leaving the spinal cord unfolded in the vertebral canal.

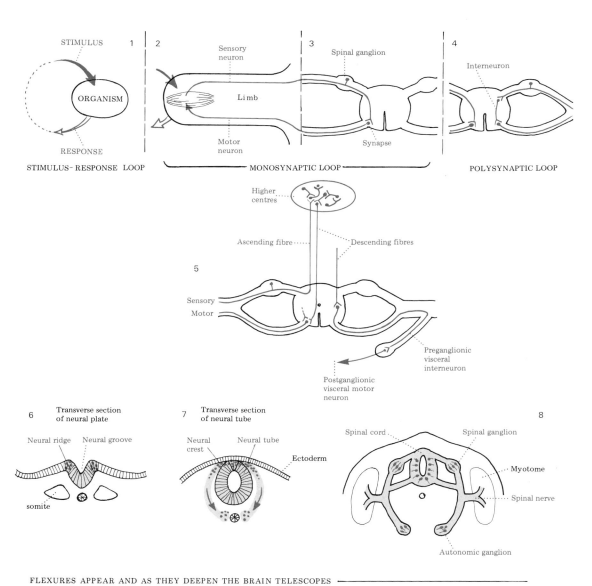

1 STIMULUS-RESPONSE LOOP

STIMULUS

ORGANISM

RESPONSE

2 — MONOSYNAPTIC LOOP — **3**

Sensory neuron

Limb

Motor neuron

Spinal ganglion

Synapse

4 POLYSYNAPTIC LOOP

Interneuron

5

Higher centres

Ascending fibre

Descending fibres

Sensory

Motor

Preganglionic visceral interneuron

Postganglionic visceral motor neuron

6 Transverse section of neural plate

Neural ridge Neural groove

somite

7 Transverse section of neural tube

Neural crest Neural tube

Ectoderm

8

Spinal cord Spinal ganglion

Myotome

Spinal nerve

Autonomic ganglion

FLEXURES APPEAR AND AS THEY DEEPEN THE BRAIN TELESCOPES

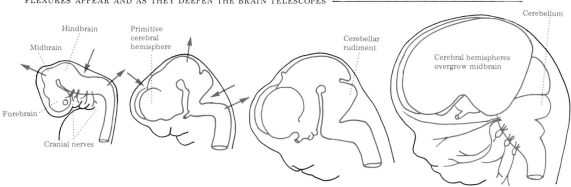

Hindbrain

Midbrain

Primitive cerebral hemisphere

Forebrain

Cranial nerves

Cerebellar rudiment

Cerebellum

Cerebral hemispheres overgrow midbrain

123

The neural tube and neural crest

Chorda-mesoderm, represented by the notochordal plate and paraxial mesoderm, exerts neuralizing and mesodermalizing effects (p. 24) on the overlying ectoderm and induces the formation of *neural plate* and *neural crest*. The epithelium of the neural plate is made up of mitotically active cells, so-called *ventricular cells*, which are characterized by abundant free polysomes and a poorly developed cytomembrane system. By the *neural tube* stage, the epithelium has become pseudo-stratified and has three nuclear zones. Next to the lumen and separated from it only by an *internal limiting membrane* is a *mitotic zone* containing the nuclei of rounded-up dividing cells. After division, the daughter cells extend their cytoplasm peripherally and their nuclei move away from the internal limiting membrane and enter a *resting zone*. As a preliminary to the next division, the nuclei move further from the internal limiting membrane and enter an outer zone where they synthesize DNA. Meanwhile, the cytoplasmic processes of the ventricular cells have extended beyond this *synthetic zone* and formed a nuclei-sparse *marginal layer* bounded by an *external limiting membrane*. The nuclei with replicated DNA, however, re-enter and pass through the resting zone, approaching the internal limiting membrane before they divide.

These undulating movements of nuclei within the *ventricular layer* are commonly referred to as *elevator movements* or *interkinetic migration*. Some of the progeny of dividing cells leave the ventricular layer without synthesizing DNA and become *neuroblasts* as they begin to develop the rough polysome-bearing endoplasmic reticulum which is characteristic of neurons. These neuroblasts accumulate in an *intermediate layer*, between the ventricular and marginal layers. Later, other daughter cells accumulate in a *subventricular layer* between the ventricular and intermediate layers. Some of the subventricular cells divide to form neuroblasts, others to form *glioblasts* which differentiate into the large-celled connective tissue of the central nervous system—the *macroglia*—astrocytes and oligodendrocytes. In contrast, the small-celled connective tissue—the *microglia*—is derived from mesenchyme, probably of neural crest origin. The cells which remain in the ventricular layer gradually reduce their mitotic activity and differentiate into ependymal cells.

The derivatives of the intermediate and subventricular layers form most of the *grey matter* of the CNS. The *white matter* is formed from myelin-forming glioblasts associated with certain neurites (processes of neuroblasts) of the marginal and subventricular layers. The wall of the neural tube remains thin at the *roof* and *floor plates*. Laterally it thickens as the intermediate layer forms two distinct masses—a *dorsal (alar) lamina* and a *ventral (basal) lamina*. As they enlarge, the masses project into the central canal and a longitudinal groove—the *sulcus limitans*—appears between them. Within the laminae, neuroblasts become multipolar as they develop a number of neurites. Most become dendrites but one elongates to form an axon. The tip of the axon divides and makes cell-membrane contacts—*synapses*—with other cells. Axons from alar neuroblasts remain within the nervous system and synapse with other neurons in both laminae. Axons from some basal neuroblasts are induced to grow beyond the confines of the neural tube, as the ventral roots of spinal nerves, to synapse with the subneural apparatus of muscle fibres or with developing autonomic neurons.

Neural Tube Histogenesis

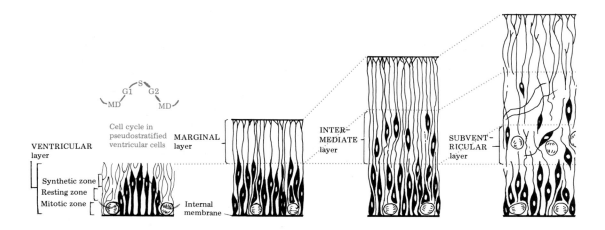

124

Neural crest

In the process of neural tube formation the *neural ridges* meet and form a midline wedge which roofs in and closes the tube. The remaining neural ridge tissue on each side forms a *neural crest* which is initially a continuous longitudinal column in the angle between neural tube and surface ectoderm. Migration of neural crest cells then occurs. Some cells destined to form *neural tissue* stop dorsolateral to the neural tube and form a series of primordia for the *spinal* and *cranial sensory ganglia*; others stop ventrolateral to the neural tube and form *sympathetic ganglia* and the *suprarenal medulla*; yet others pass into head mesenchyme or into the mesentery with viscera, and in those sites form *parasympathetic ganglia* or network of *ganglionic neurons*. Whether a particular cell becomes adrenergic or cholinergic depends upon the microenvironment in which it finds itself.

In the *spinal ganglia*, neural crest cells form bipolar neuroblasts whose peripheral and central processes complete the dorsal roots of spinal nerves. The peripheral processes reach and run with the outgrowing ventral root fibres to form mixed spinal nerves. Thence, the peripheral processes extend out and form receptor endings in the various body tissues. The central processes enter the neural tube and travel in the marginal layer to synapse with neurons at different levels in both laminae. The central and peripheral processes of the primitive bipolar neuroblasts fuse near their cell body to form the unipolar neurons of spinal ganglia. Neurons of some of the cranial sensory ganglia are also derived from neural crest cells but the neurons of others are derived from placodes (p. 73).

Neural crest tissue, which accompanies the migrating autonomic neuroblasts, differentiates into masses of sympathochromaffin cells which flank the abdominal aorta. Of these, the largest forms the suprarenal medulla while others persist for a while as *paraganglia* but many degenerate soon after birth. The *satellite cells* of ganglionic neurons (capsular cells) and of peripheral axonal processes (Schwann cells) are derived from the neural crest. When a Schwann cell is invaginated by a single axon of a certain diameter and with one of several types of peripheral termination, its plasma membrane spirals around the axon and forms an early segment of myelin sheath. (Myelin sheaths in the central nervous system form in a similar manner from the plasma membranes of processes of macroglial cells. Myelination begins near the cell body of a neuron and spreads peripherally. Growth in axonal diameter and myelin sheath thickness is generally completed within a system at about the same time as it becomes fully functional but growth in length continues until the innervated part ceases to grow.)

Neural crest tissue is also held to form the intracapsular cells of encapsulated sensory nerve endings, skin elements, including melanocytes and pigment cells, and the dental papillae and odontoblasts. It contributes to head mesenchyme in general but particularly to the facial prominences and pharyngeal arches. There it forms connective tissue elements as diverse as the skeleton, the stroma of endocrine and exocrine glands and the musculoadventitial walls of derivatives of the aortic arches. The calcitonin-producing cells of the ultimobranchial body and type I and type II cells of the carotid body are also derived from the neural crest. The optic vesicles, nasal placodes and Rathke's pouch may represent its anterior extremity and give rise to neural crest cells during development. Finally, the neural crest gives rise, in part at least, to the leptomeninges.

THE SPINAL CORD AND NERVES

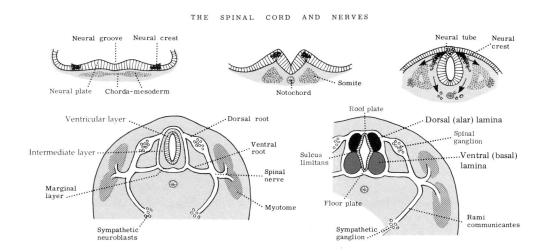

The meninges and spinal cord

The meninges

Surrounding the developing neural tube is a loose tissue—the *primitive meninx*. In the spinal region it is derived mainly from the sclerotomes, but partly from neural crest. In the cranial region it is derived from mixed head mesenchyme. The innermost cells of the primitive meninx, probably of neural crest origin, form the vascular pia mater. The outermost cells are initially indistinguishable from those of the blastemal vertebrae and membranous vault. Later, vascular channels appear and separate the spinal dura mater from perichondrium and, at the sites of the dural venous sinuses, the meningeal layer from the endosteal layer of the cerebral dura mater. The intermediate tissue cavitates and forms arachnoid trabeculae and the ligamentum denticulatum. In the *spinal region* the arachnoid mater is formed by delamination from the inner surface of the dura mater. In the *cranial region* it is more closely associated with the pia mater. At three sites the roof plate and overlying pia mater of the hindbrain break down, thus establishing communications between the cavities of the brain and the subarachnoid space; cerebrospinal fluid can then circulate. At first the spinal cord is co-extensive with the vertebral canal but in later antenatal and postnatal development, due to differential growth rates and caudal degeneration, it retreats up the canal. Cavitation of the intermediate tissue leaves an extensive subarachnoid space in the wake of the retreating cord.

The spinal cord

The early CNS—the *neuraxis*—is co-extensive with the notochord and, from within out, consists of ventricular, subventricular, intermediate and marginal layers. At this stage and throughout the length of the neuraxis, the cell bodies—*somata*—of neuroblasts are deeply placed in the subventricular and intermediate layers while their processes—*neurites*—are superficially placed in the marginal layer. The somata of neuroblasts are arranged in alar and basal laminae separated by a sulcus limitans. While it is modified in the subsequent development of the brain, this generalized arrangement persists in the spinal cord so that *spinal grey matter* (neuronal somata, dendrites, axon terminals, synapses and glia) is confined to the subependymal position and *spinal white matter* (axon bundles, myelin sheaths and associated glia) is subpial in position.

On each side of the spinal cord four longitudinal, initially cylindrical, columns of neuroblasts are formed—two derived from the alar lamina and two from the basal lamina. With continued differentiation, growth and maturation, their cylindrical form is lost but their main derivatives can be recognized in

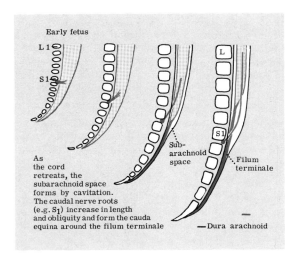

Early fetus

L1
S1

As the cord retreats, the subarachnoid space forms by cavitation. The caudal nerve roots (e.g. S_1) increase in length and obliquity and form the cauda equina around the filum terminale

Subarachnoid space

Filum terminale

Dura arachnoid

the mature cord. Each of these columns is given a name referring to the functional attributes of neurons derived from its neuroblasts. It should be noted that these neurons are usually in the minority (the majority forming interneurons of great variety), that the attribute may not be exclusive to the column and that in some situations alar neuroblasts migrate into basal laminae. Nevertheless, with these reservations, the classification is useful.

Spinal alar lamina

Each spinal alar lamina divides into a somatic afferent column adjoining the roof plate and a visceral afferent column adjoining the sulcus limitans. These columns are called 'afferent' because some of their neurons receive the synaptic terminals of some of the fibres (central processes) of primary sensory neurons which enter the CNS. Other primary afferent fibres project beyond the alar and reach the basal lamina while yet others ascend in the dorsal part of the marginal zone, providing collateral branches to the spinal grey matter as they ascend to their final destination—the gracile and cuneate nuclei in the hindbrain.

Somatic afferent column

The dorsal alar neuroblasts which form a somatic afferent column of interneurons gradually mature into most of the dorsal column (or 'horn') of the adult spinal grey matter. These neuroblasts receive the synaptic terminals of sensory neurons which convey information from somatopleuric structures (exteroceptive information from skin, proprioceptive information from striated muscle, tendon, joint capsule and fascia, and nociceptive information from all these tissues).

Visceral afferent column

The ventral neuroblasts of the alar lamina form a smaller visceral afferent column of interneurons. These neuroblasts receive the terminals of sensory neurons which convey interoceptive, including nociceptive, information from splanchnopleuric (visceral) structures and from the blood vessels and glands of the somatopleure. This column contributes to the intermediate grey matter of the mature cord.

The axons of some alar neuroblasts are involved in intra- or intersegmental local reflex loops, others invade the marginal layer and form intersegmental fibres and polysynaptic tracts to higher centres, while other long ascending or descending fibres form tracts in the developing nervous system. Many of these fibres acquire myelin sheaths so that the marginal layer is transformed into white matter. Some cross the midline in the floor plate and form the ventral white commissure of the cord. Some grow into the basal lamina.

Spinal basal lamina

Each spinal basal lamina, like an alar lamina, differentiates into two columns. These are the somatic efferent column adjoining the floor plate and the visceral efferent column adjoining the sulcus limitans. These columns are called 'efferent' because they are the source of fibres which leave the CNS.

Somatic efferent column

The ventral cells of the basal lamina form a somatic efferent column characterized by motor neurons. The axons of their neuroblasts grow out into the ventral roots and innervate striated muscle of myotomic and somatopleuric origin. Some of these neuroblasts form large multipolar neurons with large-diameter axons which supply extrafusal, somatic muscle fibres. Others form small multipolar neurons with axons of small diameter which supply the intrafusal muscle fibres of muscle spindles. The majority, however, form interneurons including the inhibitory neurons of Renshaw. Collectively, the somatic efferent cells develop into the ventral grey column (or 'horn') of the adult cord. The large neurons become grouped into subcolumns, particularly in the limb enlargements: these are related to different groups of musculature.

Visceral efferent column

The dorsal cells of the basal lamina form a visceral efferent column of interneurons. The axons of these neuroblasts grow out as preganglionic fibres which leave a ventral ramus in a white (myelinated) ramus communicans to reach a developing sympathetic ganglion, where they synapse with sympathetic neuroblasts. The postganglionic axons of the sympathetic neuroblasts either re-enter a spinal nerve in a grey (unmyelinated) ramus communicans, to be distributed to smooth muscle and secretory cells of somatopleuric origin, or pursue a direct (perivascular) course to smooth muscle and glands of splanchnopleuric origin. Axons pursue both of these courses to innervate adipose tissue. With the development of the limb enlargements of the spinal cord, the visceral efferent column becomes confined to the thoracolumbar sympathetic outflow (first thoracic to second lumbar spinal segments) and the sacral part (second to fourth segments) of the craniosacral parasympathetic outflow. Together the afferent and efferent visceral columns form much of the intermediate grey matter of the adult cord, the surface of which projects as a lateral 'horn' in the thoracic region of the cord.

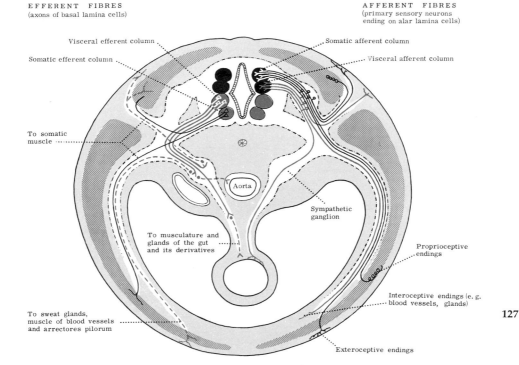

The cranial neural tube and neural crest

Whereas the generalized arrangement of the neuraxis persists in its caudal part which forms the spinal cord, it is modified in its cranial part which forms the brain. There, while some subventricular cells remain deeply placed (subependymal), others, mainly from the alar lamina, migrate through the intermediate layer into the marginal layer and thus become superficially placed. Those not migrating beyond the middle of the marginal layer differentiate into nuclei which lie between or are traversed by interweaving tracts of white matter. The vast majority, however, invade the roof plate of the brain, become virtually subpial in position and form a primitive *cortical plate*, a new zone of cell division and differentiation from which is derived superficial grey matter. Thus in the forebrain it forms the cerebral cortex, in the midbrain the colliculi (corpora quadrigemina), and in the hindbrain the cerebellar cortex.

The primary sensory neurons of the cranium are derived from neural crest or placodal tissues. The cranial neural crest forms trigeminal, acousticofacial, glossopharyngeal, vagal and transient occipital primordial ganglia. It also forms the primordial cranial autonomic ganglia (parasympathetic neuroblasts and supporting cells). It is probably also represented by Rathke's pouch, by the nasal placodes, by the optic vesicles and by a group of cells incorporated in the hindbrain which extend rostrally to form the mesencephalic nucleus of the trigeminal nerve. All the supporting cells of the definitive sensory ganglia are derived from neural crest, as are all the neurons of the superior ganglia of the glossopharyngeal and vagus nerves and some of the neurons of the tri-

geminal and geniculate ganglia (general somatic afferent). Other neurons are derived from the epibranchial placodes (V, VII, IX and X) and the otic placode of each side. Thus neuroblasts in neural crest and placodal tissues, and in the olfactory placode which forms olfactory epithelium, differentiate into the primary sensory neurons of the cranium. Their central processes provide the input at the cranial level and discharge on interneurons. The olfactory bulbs and optic nerves are forebrain derivatives and thus part of the CNS.

The brain stem

The midbrain and those parts of the hindbrain called the pons and medulla oblongata together constitute the *brain stem*, a term which thus excludes the cerebellar part of the hindbrain.

The alar and basal laminae and sulcus limitans are continued throughout the brain stem. As in the spinal cord, the laminae differentiate into somatic and visceral columns. However, in addition to general columns, which are continuous and homologous with those of the spinal cord, special columns differentiate in association with the pharyngeal arch nerves and the vestibulocochlear nerve. These special columns are limited to the medulla oblongata and pons of the hindbrain.

In the hindbrain, the roof plate is expanded and the laminae lie alongside each other in the floor of the fourth ventricle. Furthermore, cells migrate, from the lateral part of each alar lamina, ventrally and rostrally as a bulbopontine extension. The derivatives of this extension are found ventrolateral to the basal lamina derivatives and comprise the olivary, reticular and arcuate nuclei in the medulla oblongata, and the scattered pontine nuclei in the ventral part of the

Neurohistogenesis

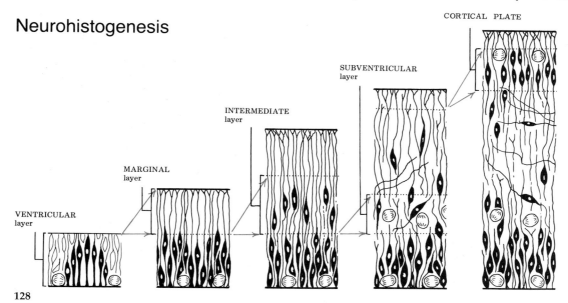

CORTICAL PLATE

SUBVENTRICULAR layer

INTERMEDIATE layer

MARGINAL layer

VENTRICULAR layer

Midbrain and Hindbrain Derivatives of Alar and Basal Laminae

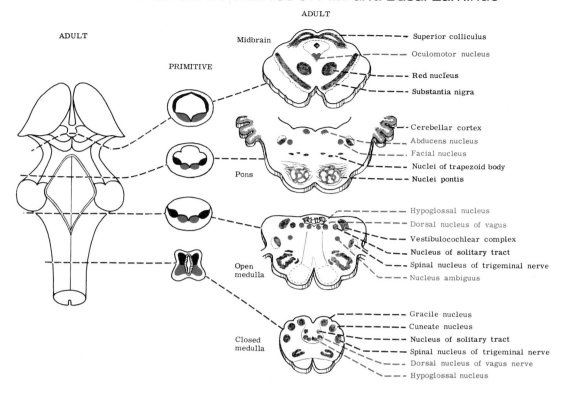

ADULT

ADULT

PRIMITIVE

Midbrain
- Superior colliculus
- Oculomotor nucleus
- Red nucleus
- Substantia nigra

Pons
- Cerebellar cortex
- Abducens nucleus
- Facial nucleus
- Nuclei of trapezoid body
- Nuclei pontis

Open medulla
- Hypoglossal nucleus
- Dorsal nucleus of vagus
- Vestibulocochlear complex
- Nucleus of solitary tract
- Spinal nucleus of trigeminal nerve
- Nucleus ambiguus

Closed medulla
- Gracile nucleus
- Cuneate nucleus
- Nucleus of solitary tract
- Spinal nucleus of trigeminal nerve
- Dorsal nucleus of vagus nerve
- Hypoglossal nucleus

pons. Finally, alar lamina cells migrate to form the cortex of the cerebellum and the nuclei in its roof. The remaining parts of the alar laminae and the basal laminae of the hindbrain form the nuclei in the floor of the fourth ventricle, including the dorsal part of the pons.

In the midbrain the alar laminae form the nuclei of the dorsal tectum and invade the roof plate, while the basal laminae form some nuclei in the ventral tegmentum and invade the floor plate. In the tegmentum, however, the red nuclei, the substantia nigra and reticular nuclei are formed from alar lamina cells which have migrated ventrally.

On inspection, the sulcus limitans appears to continue into the forebrain as the hypothalamic sulcus. On this basis some consider that the hypothalamic nuclei are derived from basal lamina. However, with some neuroendocrine exceptions, hypothalamic neurons behave like alar lamina cells and their axons remain within the nervous system. Others thus consider it preferable to regard almost all forebrain grey matter as derived from alar lamina and the sulcus limitans as ending with the midbrain.

The brain stem

Cranial alar lamina

As in the spinal cord, the cells of the alar laminae of the brain stem form interneurons. Each alar lamina differentiates into four columns. General somatic and visceral afferent columns continue upwards from the columns of the spinal cord and subserve similar functions. Between these columns a *special visceral afferent* column differentiates in the centre of the alar lamina. Its neuroblasts receive the terminals of sensory neurons which convey information from the taste buds (pharyngeal endoderm). Between the general somatic afferent column and the roof plate a *special somatic afferent* column differentiates in the most lateral part of the alar lamina. Its neuroblasts receive the terminals of sensory neurons which convey information from the organs of equilibration and hearing.

Cranial basal lamina

Three columns differentiate in each cranial basal lamina in the brain stem. Somatic and general visceral efferent columns continue upwards from the columns of the spinal cord and subserve similar functions. Between these columns a *special visceral efferent (branchiomotor)* column differentiates in the centre of the basal lamina. The axons of its neuroblasts grow out of the brain and innervate the striated special visceral (branchial) muscles of the pharyngeal arches.

Columns in the brain stem

At first, the various cell columns are continuous throughout the brain stem. Later, they break up into serially arranged masses of cells (nuclei) associated with individual cranial nerves.

Somatic efferent column

The upward continuation of the somatic efferent columns of the spinal cord form the cranial somatic efferent columns on either side of the midline floor plate. The nuclei derived from these columns contain motor neurons whose axons grow out in nerves, homologous with ventral roots, to supply striated muscle derived from myotomes or their homologues. Axons from the hypoglossal nucleus grow out to occipital myotomes which form the musculature of the tongue. Axons from the abducent nucleus grow out to the ventral part of the maxillomandibular condensation of mesenchyme, which at this stage lies lateral to the pons. The ventral part forms the lateral rectus muscle. At first the trochlear nucleus is also in the pons but later it migrates into the midbrain. Its axons grow out to the dorsal part of the maxillomandibular condensation of mesenchyme which forms the superior oblique muscle. The rostral part of the column forms most of the oculomotor complex in the midbrain. Its axons grow out to the premandibular condensation of mesenchyme which forms the other extrinsic eye muscles.

Special visceral efferent column

The cells of the basal lamina between the somatic efferent and general visceral efferent columns form a special visceral efferent (*branchiomotor*) column. The nuclei derived from it contain motor neurons whose axons supply striated special visceral (pharyngeal arch) muscle via nerves V, VII, IX, X and XI. The motor nuclei of the last three nerves form a complex. The rostral part of the complex migrates laterally and forms the nucleus ambiguus. The caudal part retains its primitive position and forms the spinal nucleus of the accessory nerve. Axons from this complex grow out in the glossopharyngeal, vagus (cranial root of the accessory) and accessory (spinal root) nerves. They supply the third and subsequent pharyngeal arch mesenchyme which forms the musculature of the pharynx, larynx and cranial half of oesophagus, and the postpharyngeal mesenchyme which forms the sternomastoid and trapezius muscles. Axons from the facial nucleus grow out to supply the second pharyngeal arch mesenchyme which forms the muscles of facial expression. Subsequently, the facial nucleus migrates around the abducens nucleus into its definitive position so that the root of the facial nerve is looped around the abducens nucleus. Axons from the motor nucleus of the trigeminal nerve grow out in the motor root and run with the mandibular division of the nerve to supply the first pharyngeal arch mesenchyme which forms the muscles of mastication. Palatine muscles' supply is mixed (p. 75).

General visceral efferent column

The upward continuation of the visceral efferent column of the spinal cord forms the cranial general visceral column which adjoins the sulcus limitans. The nuclei derived from the general visceral efferent column contain interneurons whose axons grow out as preganglionic fibres to synapse in parasympathetic ganglia, or mural visceral networks, with parasympathetic neurons of neural crest origin. The postganglionic fibres supply smooth muscle or cardiac muscle or glandular tissue. Axons from the large-celled part of the dorsal nucleus of the vagus grow out in the vagus nerve and cranial root of the accessory nerve to synapse with parasympathetic neurons in or near the walls of the foregut, the midgut and their derivatives, and the heart. Axons from the inferior salivatory nucleus grow out in the glossopharyngeal nerve to synapse with parasympathetic neurons in the otic ganglion which supply the parotid gland. Axons from the superior salivatory nucleus grow out in the facial nerve to synapse with parasympathetic neurons in the submandibular and the pterygopalatine ganglia which supply the submandibular and sublingual and other oral glands and the nasal, nasopharyngeal, palatine and lacrimal glands. The Edinger–Westphal nucleus in the midbrain migrates to the head of the oculomotor complex. Its axons grow out in the oculomotor nerve to synapse with parasympathetic neurons in the ciliary ganglion which supply the smooth intrinsic muscles of the eye (iris and ciliary body).

General visceral afferent column

The upward continuation of the visceral afferent column of the spinal cord forms the cranial general visceral afferent column which adjoins the sulcus limitans and is represented by the small-celled part of the dorsal nucleus of the vagus. Its neuroblasts receive the synaptic terminals of primary sensory neurons in the inferior ganglia of the glossopharyngeal and the vagus nerves which convey general interoceptive information from the foregut, midgut and their derivatives, and the heart. The nucleus of the solitary tract is probably also involved.

Special visceral afferent column

The cells of the alar lamina between the general visceral and general somatic afferent columns form a special visceral afferent column which is represented by the nucleus of the solitary tract. Its neuroblasts receive the terminals of sensory neurons in the geniculate ganglion of the facial nerve and the inferior ganglia of the glossopharyngeal and vagus nerves. They receive information from taste buds derived from the first, third and subsequent arch endoderm of the tongue, palate, oropharynx and epiglottis.

General somatic afferent column

The upward continuation of the somatic afferent column of the spinal cord forms the cranial general somatic afferent column which is represented in part by the main sensory nucleus and the spinal nucleus of the trigeminal nerve. Their neuroblasts receive the

terminals of sensory neurons in the trigeminal ganglion, the mesencephalic nucleus of the trigeminal nerve, the superior ganglia of the glossopharyngeal and vagus nerves. They receive proprioceptive information from the muscles of mastication (first arch), of the tongue (occipital myotomes), of the orbit (premandibular and maxillomandibular mesenchyme) and, possibly, of facial expression (second arch) via the mesencephalic nucleus. They receive exteroceptive information from the skin and ectodermal mucous membrane of the head, via the ophthalmic division (eye and frontonasal prominences) the maxillary division (maxillary prominence) and the mandibular division (mandibular prominence) of the trigeminal nerve. Additional exteroceptive information from the external ear comes via the diminutive auricular branch of the vagus and the communicating branch of the glossopharyngeal nerves. The large gracile and cuneate nuclei, which receive (amongst many others) the synaptic terminals of dorsal white column fibres conveying a massive, highly discriminative, exteroceptive and proprioceptive input from spinal levels, must also be classified as general somatic afferent.

Special somatic afferent column

The most laterally placed cells of the alar lamina form the special somatic afferent column which is represented by the vestibulocochlear complex. Its neuroblasts receive the terminals of bipolar sensory neurons in the vestibular ganglion and the spiral ganglion of the cochlea.

The Brain Stem

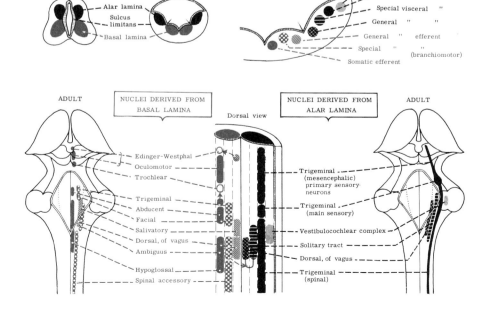

The brain

By the 7-somite stage, the neural groove has closed between the fourth and sixth somites. Cranial to the fourth somite, the expanded neural plate forms the fiddle-shaped primordial brain. The wide anterior segment is the future *prosencephalon* (forebrain). A depression near its lateral edge is the optic sulcus. The intermediate narrow segment is the future *mesencephalon* (midbrain). The posterior wide segment, continuous with the neural tube, is the future hindbrain or *rhombencephalon* (named from the rhomboidal shape which its cavity—the fourth ventricle—assumes). By the 20-somite stage, closure of the neural groove has spread and the anterior neuropore has closed, completing the primary brain vesicles. The prosencephalon, mesencephalon and rhombencephalon are now tubular structures, each containing a dilatation of the central canal. On each side the cavity of the prosencephalon opens into an optic vesicle which has grown out from the optic sulcus. At this stage the neural tube conforms with the general 'comma' shape of the embryo and has a marked primary embryonic curve. This becomes compound when a ventral flexure (cervical) appears between the rhombencephalon and the spinal cord. Another ventral flexure appears in the mesencephalon, and a dorsal flexure (pontine) follows in the rhombencephalon. Later another dorsal flexure (telencephalic) appears in the prosencephalon.

Rhombencephalon

The hindbrain of a late somite embryo shows a series of transient surface elevations (the neuromeres) which contain its differentiating efferent nuclei (IV, V, VI, VII, IX and X). At this stage the facial nucleus is rostral to the abducens nucleus but later it migrates dorsally, caudally and then ventrally into its definitive position. The trochlear nucleus migrates rostrally from the region of the isthmus—the narrow segment adjoining the mesencephalon. Meanwhile, as the pontine flexure develops, the roof plate becomes thinned, and the cavity dilates to form the diamond-shaped fourth ventricle. Its caudal and cranial angles continue into the central canal and the aqueduct of the midbrain. Its lateral angles wind around the side of the brain stem and form the lateral recesses. The ependymal roof is attached peripherally to a ridge of alar lamina—the rhombic lip. The caudal half of the rhombencephalon, lying between the level of the lateral recesses and the first cervical nerve roots, becomes the medulla oblongata. Its ependymal roof is reinforced by vascular pia mater and infolded rostrally to form the choroid plexus. The median and lateral apertures are formed by local resorption of these layers and permit cerebrospinal fluid from the ventricle to pervade the subarachnoid space. The cranial half of the rhombencephalon forms the pons. The cells of the cranial part of the rhombic lip and of the adjoining alar lamina proliferate to form the cerebellar rudiment (p. 140).

Mesencephalon

The midbrain vesicle grows much more slowly than adjacent parts, becoming relatively greatly narrowed to form the aqueduct which extends between the isthmus and the forebrain vesicle. The roof and floor plates thicken as they are invaded by lamina cells and form the midline parts of the tectum and tegmentum. Most of the nuclei differentiate within the midbrain, but the trochlear nucleus migrates from the isthmus, and the mesencephalic trigeminal nucleus extends from the pons. The tectum becomes subdivided by surface depressions into superior and inferior pairs of colliculi, which are reflex, correlation and relay centres for visual and auditory information, but modulated by inputs from the spinal cord, reticular formation and cerebellar and cerebral cortices. The ventral part of the marginal layer is invaded by massive tracts of fibres which descend from the forebrain on each side and form the cerebral peduncles.

Prosencephalon

Rostral to the optic cups, the forebrain develops massive bilateral evaginations which are the primitive cerebral hemispheres. Each contains a lateral ventricle which communicates with the prosencephalic cavity (third ventricle) by an interventricular foramen. The rostral wall of the third ventricle is a thin sheet—the lamina terminalis—in which the optic chiasma and major cerebral commissures develop (p. 134). The primitive hemispheres, the lamina terminalis and the brain wall between them constitute the telencephalon (end-brain). The rest of the third ventricle and its walls constitute the diencephalon (between-brain).

Diencephalon

The third ventricle becomes laterally compressed as epithalamic, thalamic, hypothalamic and subthalamic nuclear masses appear in its lateral walls. These masses form reflex, correlation and relay centres: the epithalamus for olfactory information and the maintenance of some biorhythms mediated by the pineal gland; the thalamus for all sensory information except olfactory; and the hypothalamus for visceral and olfactory information. The hypothalamic mass continues into the floor of the ventricle, where a median diverticulum forms the rudiment of the neurohypophysis. The roof remains thin except caudally where the pineal gland, habenular nuclei and related commissures form.

Telencephalon

The corpus striatum (a primitive motor control centre) develops as a nuclear mass in the floor of each lateral ventricle. Elsewhere, the walls constitute the pallium or cortex. The hemispheres expand dorsally, caudally and, to a lesser extent, rostrally. They be-

The Brain

VENTRAL FLEXURES APPEAR
IN THE LATE-SOMITE EMBRYO

DORSAL FLEXURES APPEAR
IN THE POSTSOMITE EMBRYO

AS THEY DEEPEN
THE BRAIN TELESCOPES

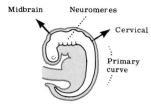

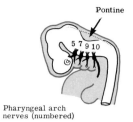

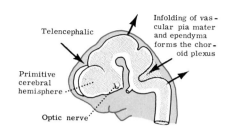

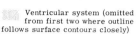

Ventricular system (omitted from first two where outline follows surface contours closely)

HEMISPHERES EXPAND AND APPROACH - THE INTERVENING MESENCHYME FORMS DURAL PARTITIONS

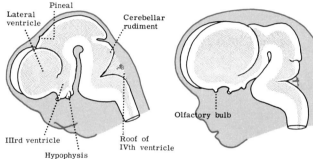

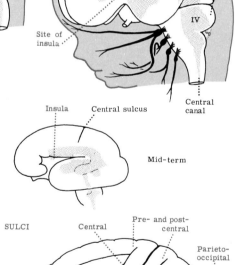

come dorsiflexed on the diencephalon and gradually grow over it and the mesencephalon. The rostral part of each hemisphere forms the frontal lobe and has an olfactory bulb on its under-surface. The caudal part curves downwards and forwards behind the developing eye and forms the temporal lobe. Later, a further backward extension forms the occipital lobe. The lateral ventricle extends into these lobes as its anterior, inferior and posterior horns. At first, the surfaces of the hemispheres are smooth, but, as growth proceeds, the pallium is thrown into a number of complex folds or gyri with intervening sulci. The groove between the frontal and temporal lobes forms the stem of the lateral sulcus. As the hemisphere grows, the cortex covering the corpus striatum remains relatively static, and is overgrown by a series of opercula from the surrounding cortex. The buried cortex forms the insula, and the opercula meet at the posterior ramus of the lateral sulcus. Other sulci may be limiting (infolding around the 'margins' of a so-called functional area) or axial (infolding within a 'functional area') or merely reflect growth within a confined space and have no functional significance.

It should be noted that while the concepts of 'centres' and 'functional areas' are useful at an introductory level, they do not stand up to sophisticated analysis.

The forebrain

Like the roof of the primitive fourth ventricle, the roof of most of the third ventricle and a curved strip in the medial wall of the lateral ventricle do not develop nervous tissue, but become membranous. In these regions vascular pia mater overlies the ependymal lining of the ventricle and forms the *primitive tela choroidea*. Invaginations into the ventricles form *choroid plexuses*. The site of invagination into a lateral ventricle is termed the *choroid fissure*. At this stage a horizontal section through the diencephalon and telencephalon, caudal to the interventricular foramen, shows the diencephalon with the developing thalamus and hypothalamus in its lateral wall, and the telencephalon separated from it by the primitive meninx. In the floor of the telencephalon is the developing corpus striatum. Apart from these subependymal nuclei, neuroblasts from the subventricular layer invade the marginal layer and form a cortical plate which differentiates into three main areas of superficial cortical grey matter. Of these, two are initially associated with olfaction. The central processes of primary sensory neurons in the olfactory mucous membrane become grouped into bundles—the olfactory nerves. These grow into the telencephalon at the future olfactory bulbs and make synaptic contact with mitral and other varieties of neuroblast. The axons of the mitral cells grow back in the olfactory tract which divides into lateral and medial roots. The medial root runs to a strip of cortex immediately dorsal to the choroidal fissure—the *archipallium* (hippocampal cortex). The lateral root runs to an area of cortex lateral to the anterior part of the striatum—the *palaeopallium* (piriform cortex). Between these primitive olfactory cortices is the *neopallium* which deals with motor control, with sensory information relayed from the diencephalic nuclei and with higher thought processes. It expands enormously during subsequent development. The olfactory input to archi- and palaeopallial structures should not be over-stressed. Both develop massive interconnections with neopallial cortical areas, the hypothalamus, thalamus, reticular formation and other centres in the brain stem. Thus they become involved in polydimensional perception, total environmental orientation, the establishment of memory traces and the planning of executive commands for complex behavioural responses.

The fibres of the interneurons which make up much of the white matter of the forebrain are of three kinds: *commissural fibres* cross the midline and bring the two sides into communication, *association fibres* connect different areas of the same side and bring them into communication, while *projection fibres* connect the forebrain with the brain stem and spinal cord.

Commissural and association fibres

Cortical and other areas become connected with the opposite side by *commissural* axons. Many of these cross the midline in the *lamina terminalis*. Its lowest part is invaded by decussating axons from the ganglion cells of the retina and forms the *optic chiasma*. Above this, axons connect the piriform cortices and olfactory bulbs and form the primitive *anterior commissure*. Above, again, axons connect the hippocampal cortices and form the primitive *commissure of the fornix*. Axons connecting the neopallial cortices run mainly in the upper part of the lamina, where they form the *corpus callosum*, but they also reinforce the posterior part of the anterior commissure. Other commissures develop in the caudal part of the roof of the third ventricle in relation to the stalk of the pineal gland. Above it, axons connecting the two epithalami form the *habenular commissure*, collateral branches probably invading the pineal gland as the habenulo-pineal tract. Below it, axons connecting certain diencephalic and mesencephalic nuclei form the *posterior commissure*. Different cortical areas in the same hemisphere become connected by long and short arcuate *association* axons.

The Forebrain and its Commissures

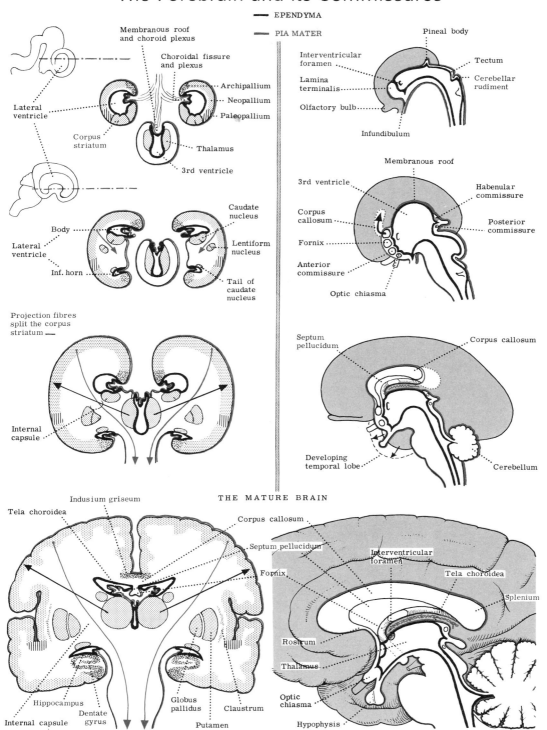

EPENDYMA
PIA MATER

Membranous roof and choroid plexus
Choroidal fissure and plexus
Archipallium
Neopallium
Paleopallium
Corpus striatum
Thalamus
3rd ventricle
Lateral ventricle

Pineal body
Interventricular foramen
Lamina terminalis
Olfactory bulb
Tectum
Cerebellar rudiment
Infundibulum

Caudate nucleus
Body
Lentiform nucleus
Lateral ventricle
Inf. horn
Tail of caudate nucleus

Membranous roof
3rd ventricle
Habenular commissure
Corpus callosum
Fornix
Posterior commissure
Anterior commissure
Optic chiasma

Projection fibres split the corpus striatum
Internal capsule

Septum pellucidum
Corpus callosum
Developing temporal lobe
Cerebellum

THE MATURE BRAIN

Indusium griseum
Tela choroidea
Corpus callosum
Septum pellucidum
Fornix
Hippocampus
Dentate gyrus
Internal capsule
Globus pallidus
Putamen
Claustrum

Interventricular foramen
Tela choroidea
Splenium
Rostrum
Thalamus
Optic chiasma
Hypophysis

135

As the neopallium expands, the corpus callosum also expands and grows back *over* the choroid fissure, forming the rostrum, genu, body and splenium of the corpus callosum. It carries an investment of pia mater with it so that a flat tunnel, lined by pia mater, extends from the transverse fissure (between the pineal gland and the splenium of the corpus callosum) forwards to the region of the interventricular foramina. The tunnel is bounded by the corpus callosum and fornix superiorly, the choroid fissure in the body of the lateral ventricle laterally and the epithelial roof of the third ventricle inferiorly. The double fold of pia mater and its contained mesenchyme form the definitive tela choroidea and carry arteries to the neighbouring choroid plexuses, and veins which, in addition to draining the plexuses, drain large volumes of deeply placed neural tissues. In its backward growth, the corpus callosum carries the commissure of the fornix on its under-surface.

As the caudal pole of the hemisphere grows downwards and forwards and forms the temporal lobe, many of the slightly curved, but almost linear, structures of the primitive hemisphere grow along a progressively more highly curved course. The lateral ventricle and corpus striatum are carried into the temporal lobe as the inferior horn, the tail of the caudate nucleus and the amygdaloid body. The hippocampal cortex and surrounding tissues (hippocampal formation) also become C-shaped as they are carried round in relation to the choroid fissure. The ventral limb of the C-shaped hippocampal formation is unaffected by the backward growth of the corpus callosum. It becomes complexly folded and forms the dentate gyrus and the cornu ammonis of the hippocampus. The dorsal limb is reduced by the encroachment of the corpus callosum to mere rudiments—the indusium griseum and the longitudinal striae.

Projection fibres

Axons projected from neopallial neuroblasts traverse the dorsal part of the corpus striatum and partially subdivide it into a superomedial (caudate) and an inferolateral (lentiform) nucleus. The lateral surfaces of the diencephalon become fused with the medial surfaces of the hemispheres within the curve of the choroid fissure. The neopallial projection axons, with axons projected from thalamic and hypothalamic neuroblasts across the fused area to the neopallium, constitute the internal capsule. This passes lateral to the body of the lateral ventricle and medial to its inferior horn. The neopallial projection axons then traverse the fused area and the cerebral peduncles to reach interneurons and motor neurons in the brain stem and spinal cord. (Virtually *all* subcortical masses of grey matter receive direct or indirect projections from neopallial neurons, modulating their transmission characteristics. In turn, reciprocal paths back to the neopallium are established.) In addition to commissural, arcuate and projection neurons, other neurons with shorter ramifying or horizontal axons develop and bring the different layers of the laminated cortex into functional relationship.

As elsewhere in the neural tube, the walls of the earliest cerebral hemispheres consist of a pseudo-stratified epithelium, within which the nuclei of ventricular cells show elevator movement or interkinetic migration. Again, as elsewhere, subventricular, intermediate and marginal layers develop outside the ventricular layer. Mature neocortical neurons, which are arranged in tangential laminae numbered from the pia inwards, are derived from subventricular neuroblasts that migrate to form a cortical plate in the superficial part of the marginal layer. The fully differentiated, immediately subpial, part of the early marginal layer forms lamina I (plexiform)—mainly neurites and associated glia, with only a sparse population of neurons. The first *cellular* laminae to differentiate from migrating neuroblasts are lamina VI (multiform) and lamina V (ganglionic). Subsequent generations of migrating neuroblasts pass *through* the territories of laminae VI and V and successively differentiate into laminae IV (internal granular), III (pyramidal) and II (external granular) from within outwards.

The Forebrain and its Commissures

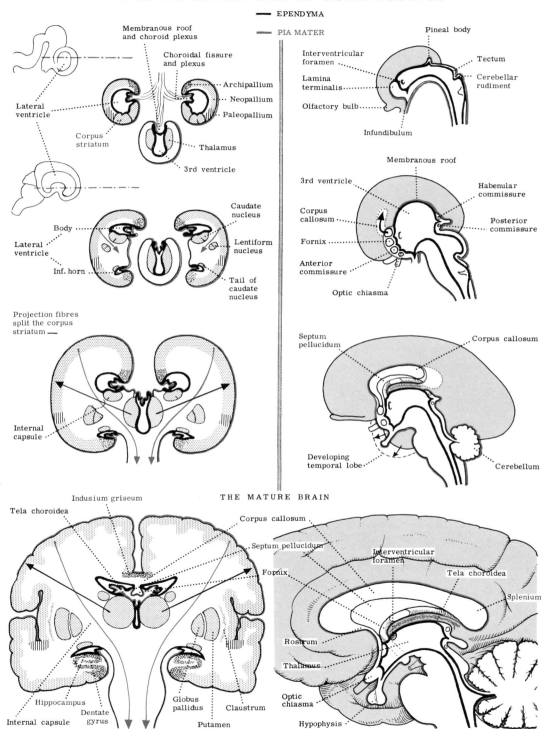

— EPENDYMA

— PIA MATER

Membranous roof and choroid plexus

Choroidal fissure and plexus

Archipallium

Neopallium

Paleopallium

Lateral ventricle

Corpus striatum

Thalamus

3rd ventricle

Caudate nucleus

Body

Lateral ventricle

Lentiform nucleus

Inf. horn

Tail of caudate nucleus

Projection fibres split the corpus striatum

Internal capsule

Interventricular foramen

Lamina terminalis

Olfactory bulb

Infundibulum

Pineal body

Tectum

Cerebellar rudiment

Membranous roof

3rd ventricle

Corpus callosum

Fornix

Anterior commissure

Optic chiasma

Habenular commissure

Posterior commissure

Septum pellucidum

Corpus callosum

Developing temporal lobe

Cerebellum

THE MATURE BRAIN

Indusium griseum

Tela choroidea

Corpus callosum

Septum pellucidum

Fornix

Interventricular foramen

Tela choroidea

Splenium

Rostrum

Thalamus

Optic chiasma

Hypophysis

Hippocampus

Dentate gyrus

Internal capsule

Globus pallidus

Claustrum

Putamen

The limbic system

The formation of the temporal lobe brings the caudal ends of the two 'primitive' cortices (the archipallium and the palaeopallium) into secondary continuity as the piriform cortex and the hippocampus (cornu ammonis and dentate gyrus). These structures are derived from neuroblasts that *border* the convex external margins of the interventricular foramen and its curved caudal extension, the choroid fissure; hence the collective name *limbic lobe* (L. *limbus* = border) or *limbic system* when its numerous connections and functional associations are included. Traced radially from the outer lip of the choroid fissure, the derived tissues show increasing complexity of structure, and this remains evident even after the complicated infolding of layers has occurred. Near the fissure, and most elementary in structure, lies the *dentate gyrus*, followed by the more highly ordered *cornu ammonis*, then progressing through the still further differentiated regions of the *subiculum*, to finally merge with fully developed *neopallium*.

At first, the *primitive fornix* consists only of commissural fibres connecting the hippocampal cortices. Soon, other axons from hippocampal neuroblasts traverse the lateral part of the fornix to reach diencephalic and other nuclei of the same side. When the corpus callosum grows backwards, the commissural part of the fornix becomes confined to an area above the ependymal roof of the third ventricle. With the formation of the temporal lobe, the backward growth of the corpus callosum and the reduction of the dorsal part of the hippocampal formation, the lateral fibres pursue a long, curved course. On each side they leave the medial edge of the hippocampal formation, in the floor of the inferior horn, and form a hippocampal fimbria. From the fimbriae they traverse the right and left crura of the fornix. The crura are joined across the midline by the commissural fibres and fuse at the body of the fornix. The fornix divides again above the interventricular foramina, and homolateral fibres descend in the right and left columns to reach and terminate in septal, hypothalamic and reticular nuclei. Between the expanding corpus callosum and fornix, lamina terminalis tissue and paraterminal archipallial septal cortex become attenuated and form two thin paramedian laminae—the *septum pellucidum*.

After fusion between the telencephalon and diencephalon, the expanding thalami enroach on the third and lateral ventricles. In the third ventricle, fusion produces a variable interthalamic adhesion. In each lateral ventricle, the thalamus forms the medial part of the floor of the body and, in it, is separated from the corpus striatum by a bundle of axons which project from the amygdaloid body and pass rostrally to the piriform cortex and the hypothalamus as the *stria terminalis*. This, too, becomes C-shaped as the temporal lobe grows. In the angle between the lateral wall and roof of the third ventricle, axons pass between the piriform cortex and the epithalamus and habenular commissure in the *stria medullaris thalami*. Neither this tract nor the *medial forebrain bundle*, which interconnects piriform cortex, hypothalamus and reticular nuclei, is affected by the growth of the temporal lobe.

The parts primitively concerned with olfaction were for long grouped together as the so-called rhinencephalon (smell-brain). In man, however, only the piriform cortex (palaeopallium) seems to be concerned with conscious olfactory experience. With the archipallial component and amygdaloid body, projections to the hypothalamus, epithalamus, hypothalamic projections to the cingulate gyrus and the cingulate gyrus itself, the subiculum and parahippocampal gyrus, and their numerous neocortical interconnections, it forms the basis of the limbic system.

Limbic Lobe

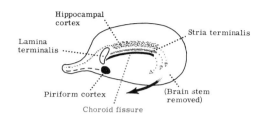

Hippocampal cortex

Lamina terminalis

Stria terminalis

Piriform cortex

(Brain stem removed)

Choroid fissure

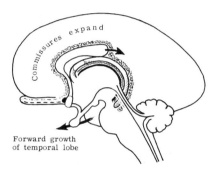

Commissures expand

Forward growth of temporal lobe

Medial surface of right hemisphere
with details of brain stem removed
for clarity

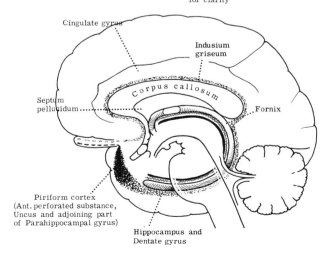

Cingulate gyrus

Indusium griseum

Corpus callosum

Septum pellucidum

Fornix

Piriform cortex
(Ant. perforated substance,
Uncus and adjoining part
of Parahippocampal gyrus)

Hippocampus and
Dentate gyrus

The cerebellum

The neuroblasts of the cranial part of the rhombic lip and the adjoining alar lamina proliferate to form bilateral cerebellar rudiments. At first, these project into the fourth ventricle, but soon they meet and form a dumb-bell-shaped swelling which projects externally. A *posterolateral sulcus* appears and demarcates the *flocculonodular lobe*. A *primary fissure* separates the *anterior* and *middle lobes*. Numerous less significant fissures appear and give rise to the folia of the cerebellum. The cerebellar cortex may be divided into three (overlapping) zones which receive afferent fibres from different sources. The neuroblasts of the *archicerebellum* receive equilibratory information, directly and after relay in the vestibular nuclei, from the bipolar neurons of the vestibular ganglion. The *palaeocerebellum splits the archicerebellum* into a small rostral part—the lingula—and a larger caudal part—the flocculonodular lobe. The neuroblasts of the palaeocerebellum receive tactile and proprioceptive information, after relay and perhaps directly from the unipolar neurons of the spinal and trigeminal nerves. The *neocerebellum splits the palaeocerebellum* into a rostral part, mostly the anterior lobe, and a caudal part the pyramid, uvula and tonsils. The neocerebellum forms mostly the middle lobe and receives the terminals of cerebral, tectal and olivary neuroblasts. The rostrocaudal division of the cerebellar cortex into main regions, depending upon their principal (but not exclusive) sources of afferent input, is only one method of classification. Alternative criteria result in different divisions.

Two distinct waves of migration occur from subventricular alar presumptive neuroblasts of the cranial part of the rhombic lips into the membranous roof of the fourth ventricle. One remains for a while subependymal and forms an *internal germinal layer* whilst the other forms a subpial cortical plate—the *external germinal layer*. Orderly sequences of further migration, differentiation and growth occur at both sites.

The cells of the *internal germinal layer* form three main groups of definitive neuroblasts. *Nuclear neuroblasts* remain subependymal and form the deep cerebellar ('roof') nuclei (archicerebellar-fastigial; palaeocerebellar-emboliform and globose; neocerebellar-dentate), their axons growing via the cerebellar peduncles to their destinations in motor control integrative centres throughout the brain stem and diencephalon. In contrast, *Purkinje neuroblasts* migrate superficially from the internal germinal layer to the junction of molecular and granular layers where they distribute in precisely patterned arrays, their flattened dendritic trees penetrating the molecular layer whilst their axons retain synaptic contact with neuroblasts of the deep roof nuclei. Somewhat later another superficial migration of *Golgi neuroblasts* occurs and they almost reach the Purkinje cells before developing their relatively vast dendritic and axonal arborizations.

The *external germinal layer* gives rise first to generations of *stellate* and *basket cell neuroblasts*, both differentiating in a subpial position in the future molecular layer. Soon this is followed by an intense proliferation of cortical plate cells to give a vast population of *granule cell neuroblasts*; these migrate deeply (centripetally), meeting and then passing through the Purkinje cell layer. Some remain dispersed between the somata of the Golgi neurons, but the majority form a densely packed granular layer deep to them. The granule neuroblasts migrate with their rudimentary dendrites in advance; ultimately these make synaptic contacts with incoming 'mossy' cerebellar afferents and Golgi cell axon terminals in the spherical complex cerebellar synaptic glomeruli that occupy the crevices between adjacent granule cell clusters. The tip of the elongating granule cell axon remains in the molecular layer and bifurcates at right angles, each branch growing a few millimetres in the long axis of its cerebellar folium. Collectively these branches form the parallel fibre bundles of the cortex.

The Cerebellum

1

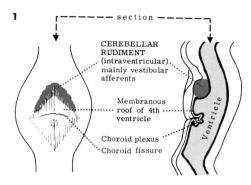

— — — — — section — — — — —

CEREBELLAR
RUDIMENT
(intraventricular).
mainly vestibular
afferents

Membranous
roof of 4th
ventricle

Choroid plexus

Choroid fissure

Ventricle

2 EXTROVERSION : Afferents from spinal cord
subdivide the vestibular area

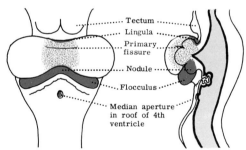

Tectum

Lingula

Primary
fissure

Nodule

Flocculus

Median aperture
in roof of 4th
ventricle

3 Further invasion and subdivision by afferents from
neopallium

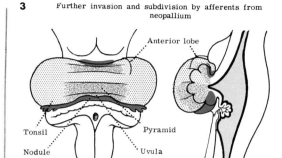

Anterior lobe

Tonsil

Nodule

Pyramid

Uvula

4 MATURE CEREBELLUM

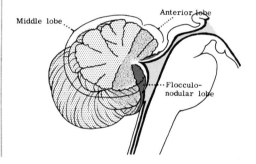

Middle lobe

Anterior lobe

Flocculo-
nodular lobe

Anomalies

While occurring less frequently than spina bifida occulta (p. 116), *spina bifida cystica* remains very common. Where the gap due to non-union of paired vertebral arches is *primary* and is wide, normally developed meninges and spinal cord may extend through it so that a sac covered with skin is seen on the surface. In a *meningocele*, only the meninges bulge through the gap; in some cases of *meningomyelocele* a normally developed cord is in the sac and may be adherent to it. Where the non-union of vertebral arches is *secondary* to defective neural tube formation, the overlying skin or skin and meninges may be absent so that the thin membrane of the sac is exposed or absent. In cases of *meningomyelocele* in this category, the thin membrane and meninges are initially intact but may be easily torn and the extruded cord is abnormal; in a *meningohydromyelocele* its central canal is distended. In a *myelocele* the neural tube has not closed and an open plate of nervous tissue is widely exposed to the surface. Lesions are most commonly associated with the posterior end of the tube (i.e. the lumbosacral region) but any part or the whole of the spine can be affected.

In the same way, contents of the cranium may herniate through large primary defects of the skull, the occipital region being the commonest site. In a *meningocele*, only the arachnoid is herniated, the dura being related to the periosteum and therefore defective and the pia following the contours of the brain. In a *meningoencephalocele*, brain and pia are also herniated, whilst in a *meningohydroencephalocele* a diverticulum from a ventricle is included.

Neurological signs are absent in uncomplicated (closed) cases of meningocele, meningomyelocele and encephalocele, and surgical repair is frequently successful. In other cases, particularly in myelocele where the exposed nervous tissue has undergone secondary degeneration and vascularization prenatally, neurological signs such as paralysis are present. Most such cases die before the age of 3 years, usually from infection of the exposed nervous tissue. Closure of the defect may be life-saving but there is no way of replacing damaged nervous tissue.

Iniencephaly is an uncommon variant of spina bifida, due to defective development of the cervical and occipital sclerotomes and the parachordal cartilages. As a result, there are defects of the squamous part of the occipital bone and of the cervical vertebrae, with prolapse of the brain through the enlarged foramen magnum.

In some cases of spina bifida cystica the spinal cord remains tethered to the skin and vertebrae at the site of the lesion and thus does not, as normally, retreat up the vertebral canal. As a result, the hindbrain is compressed in the cervical vertebral canal and plugs the foramen magnum. Cerebrospinal fluid is thus unable to escape via the fourth ventricle and distends the brain, producing *hydrocephaly*. (In cases of hydrocephaly not associated with spina bifida the common site of obstruction is the aqueduct of the midbrain, so only the lateral and third ventricles are affected.)

Both anencephaly and exencephaly are due to defective closure of the anterior end of the neural tube. In *exencephaly*, which is found only in the embryos and early fetuses, the scalp and vault of the skull fail to develop over an open but substantial mass of folded brain tissue. *Anencephaly*, which develops from exencephaly by secondary degeneration and vascularization of the exposed nerve tissue, presents in later fetuses and newborn babies which may be stillborn or short-lived: an exposed flattened mass of vascular, cystic nervous tissue sits on the base of the skull and is frequently continuous with a cervical myelocele.

In both anencephaly and open spina bifida, cerebrospinal fluid and vascular transudate are discharged into the amniotic fluid and cause hydramnios; in anencephaly the neural mechanism for swallowing is defective, which also contributes to the degree of hydramnios. The leakage of fetal blood or blood components into the amniotic fluid raises the level of α-fetoprotein above normal levels and may be detected following amniocentesis (p. 56). However, the α-fetoprotein level is raised in other conditions associated with leakage and is not raised in closed cases of spina bifida. The test is thus not particularly discriminatory and diagnosis by ultrasound is more reliable.

Spina bifida cystica and anencephaly together are amongst the commonest serious congenital conditions, in incidence being second only to congenital heart disease. Their inheritance is multifactorial. They are commoner in girls and in caucasians but regional variations in incidence exceed those of sex and race. The incidence of second affected babies in families with one affected is high, as is the incidence in the offspring of consanguineous marriages. The conditions have rarely been found in identical twin pregnancies and then only one twin has been affected. It is likely that pregnancies in which both twins have been affected have been abortive.

SPINA BIFIDA CYSTICA   PRIMARY anomalies are due to non-union of vertebral arches only

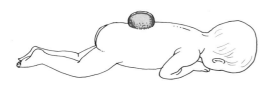

MENINGOCELE

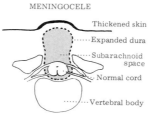

- Thickened skin
- Expanded dura
- Subarachnoid space
- Normal cord
- Vertebral body

MENINGOMYELOCELE

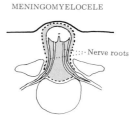

- Nerve roots

SECONDARY anomalies are those where non-union of vertebral arches is due to defective neural tube formation

MENINGOMYELOCELE

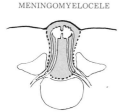

MENINGOHYDROMYELOCELE

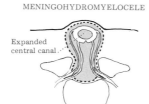

Expanded central canal

MYELOCELE

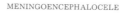
Open cord

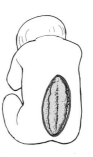

CRANIAL MENINGOCELE

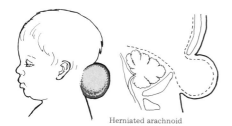

Herniated arachnoid

MENINGOENCEPHALOCELE

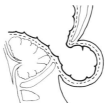

Herniated brain tissue

MENINGOHYDRO-ENCEPHALOCELE

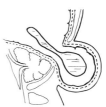

Herniated brain and ventricular lumen

INIENCEPHALY

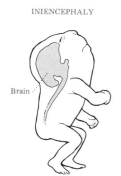

Brain

HYDROCEPHALY

Hydrocephalus
+
spina bifida
cystica

≡ Arnold—Chiari malformation

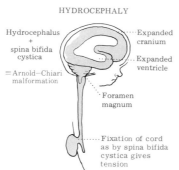

- Expanded cranium
- Expanded ventricle
- Foramen magnum
- Fixation of cord as by spina bifida cystica gives tension

EXENCEPHALY

Exposed brain

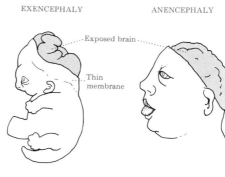

Thin membrane

ANENCEPHALY

143

The Eye

The optic vesicle induces the formation of a lens vesicle from the overlying head ectoderm and forms a double-walled optic cup. This and the adjoining optic stalk are incomplete inferiorly, where they wrap around a strand of vascular mesenchyme, at the choroidal fissure. The hyaloid artery forms in this mesenchyme and supplies the vascular capsule of the developing lens. Branches arise from the proximal part of the artery and supply the inner wall of the optic cup. The distal part and the posterior lens capsule subsequently degenerate. As the lips of the choroidal fissure fuse, the hyaloid artery becomes enclosed within the solid optic nerve as the central artery of the retina. The choroidal fissure may not close completely, resulting in a congenital cleft iris or *coloboma*. The hyaloid artery may persist and form an opacity in the vitreous body.

The margins of the optic cup extend and overlap the lens. Posterior to it, the inner wall of the cup forms the retina proper (rod and cone cells, bipolar cells, ganglionic cells, horizontal and amacrine cells and supporting elements) while the outer wall forms the pigmented layer of the retina. Anteriorly, the walls of the cup continue as the two-layered epithelium on the posterior surface of the ciliary body and iris. In the iris, optic cup cells (neural ectoderm) form the sphincter and dilator pupillae muscles. The mesenchyme surrounding the cup condenses to form an inner vascular coat—the choroid and the rest of the iris and ciliary body, including the ciliary muscle—and an outer fibrous coat—the sclera and the substantia propria of the cornea. Anterior and posterior chambers are at first separated by the anterior part of the mesenchymatous lens capsule—the pupillary membrane—which normally breaks down as term approaches but may persist. The margins of the eyelid folds fuse and remain fused, forming a closed conjunctival sac, until the fetus is viable (p. 162). The lacrimal gland arises as a series of ectodermal cords which grow from the outer part of the upper conjunctival recess (fornix) into the underlying mesenchyme. These ramify and later canalize, forming the secretory units and multiple ducts of the gland. The axons of the neuroblasts of the ganglionic layer of the retina converge on the optic papilla and grow through the neuroglial framework of the primitive optic nerve towards the lamina terminalis. There the fibres from the nasal half of each retina decussate and form the optic chiasma. The fibres of the optic tract are thus derived from the temporal half of the homolateral retina and the nasal half of the contralateral retina. They continue to grow round the side of the upper end of the midbrain (cerebral peduncles) and terminate in the developing thalamus (lateral geniculate body), the tectum (superior colliculus), and probably other diencephalic centres. The developing lenses are vulnerable to the rubella virus (German measles) and may become opaque—*congenital cataract*—resulting in blindness.

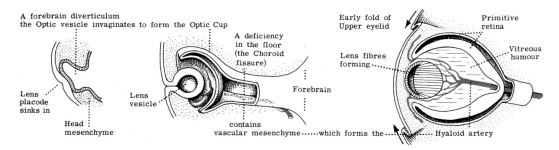

A forebrain diverticulum the Optic vesicle invaginates to form the Optic Cup

Lens placode sinks in

Head mesenchyme

Lens vesicle

A deficiency in the floor (the Choroid fissure)

Forebrain

contains vascular mesenchyme ......which forms the.... Hyaloid artery

Early fold of Upper eyelid

Lens fibres forming

Primitive retina

Vitreous humour

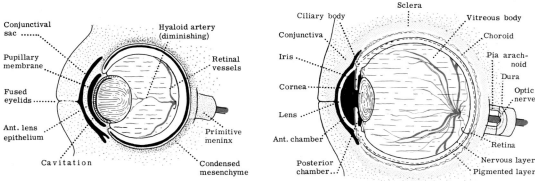

Conjunctival sac

Pupillary membrane

Fused eyelids

Ant. lens epithelium

Cavitation

Hyaloid artery (diminishing)

Retinal vessels

Primitive meninx

Condensed mesenchyme

Ciliary body

Conjunctiva

Iris

Cornea

Lens

Ant. chamber

Posterior chamber

Sclera

Vitreous body

Choroid

Pia arachnoid

Dura

Optic nerve

Retina

Nervous layer

Pigmented layer

The Ear

The pinna arises by the fusion of tubercles around the orifice of the first pharyngeal groove. The lining of the external acoustic meatus and the outer epithelium of the tympanic membrane are derived from first groove ectoderm. The dorsal recesses of the first and second endodermal pouches combine to form a common tubotympanic recess which grows towards the first groove ectoderm. As the tubotympanic recess expands around the auditory ossicles and the chorda tympani, it invests them with endoderm, continuous with that lining the walls of the recess. The endoderm also clothes the inner aspect of the tympanic membrane, which thus represents the closing membrane between the first groove and the first pouch. In this way, the recess forms the tympanic cavity proper and the auditory tube. Later extensions form the epitympanic recess and the mastoid antrum. At term, the mastoid air cells begin to develop. Meanwhile, on each side, an ectodermal placode sinks below the surface and forms an otic vesicle—the primordium of the membranous labyrinth. An early outgrowth from its medial aspect is the endolymphatic sac. The otic vesicle is related to and contributes to the acoustico-facial complex of neural crest material. After the geniculate ganglion of the facial nerve has separated from the complex, the otic vesicle and the remaining ganglionic tissue become subdivided into vestibular and cochlear parts. Three flattened diverticula arise from the dorsal (vestibular) part. Only the peripheral rims of these diverticula remain patent. They form the semicircular ducts opening off a utriculosaccular chamber. At first the anterior and posterior semi-circular ducts are in the same plane, but later the posterior duct swings laterally into its definitive position. The ventral (cochlear) part elongates, becomes coiled and forms the cochlear duct. The cells forming that part of the duct related to the basilar membrane differentiate into the rows of sensory hair cells and wide variety of supporting cells that characterize the organ of Corti. Subsequently the connections between the various parts become narrowed. Particular patches of cells in the walls of the utricle and saccule differentiate and form polarized rows of sensory hair cells with their related otolithic membrane and supporting cells; they constitute the maculae of these endolymphatic cavities. The mesenchyme surrounding the middle and internal ears chondrifies and forms the cartilaginous otic capsule. The perilymphatic space develops between the membranous labyrinth and the cartilage, and approaches the tympanic cavity at the round and oval windows. The neuroblasts of the vestibular and spiral (cochlear) ganglia are bipolar. Their peripheral processes grow into the membranous labyrinth, and end in relation to cells with hair-like processes in the dilated end (ampulla) of each semicircular duct, the utricle, the saccule and in the spiral organ of the cochlear duct. Their central processes grow back to synapse with, and convey auditory and equilibratory information to, the vestibulocochlear complex in the lateral part of the floor of the fourth ventricle. The rubella virus may affect the developing inner ear, later resulting in deaf-mutism.

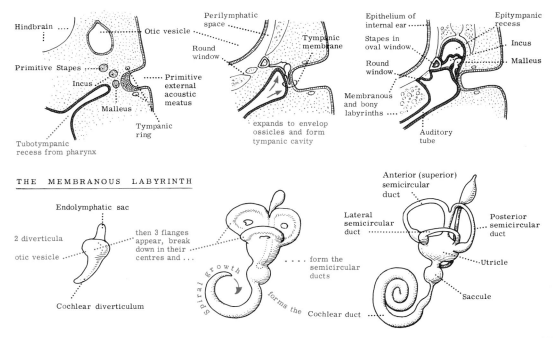

THE MEMBRANOUS LABYRINTH

The Vascular System

As the embryo becomes larger and more complex, it develops a more efficient delivery method than that provided by the fluid-filled coelomic spaces. A distinct circulatory blood vascular system brings fluids into the body and delivers them to the tissues where they give up oxygen, nutrients and some water in exchange for carbon dioxide and other waste products.

The formation of the system begins in the wall of the yolk sac which was the source of nutrients in ancestral forms, as it is in the chick. Groups of mesoderm cells form blood islands in which the cells around the outside become the lining cells—*endothelium*—of blood vessels and the cells on the inside become *primitive blood cells*. The islands link up to form a vascular network in the yolk sac wall. Meanwhile, empty vessels (containing no blood cells) form independently in the mesoderm of the connecting stalk and of the chorion, including its villi. Isolated vessels also form within the embryo and join to form continuous vessels on each side of the body.

The chorionic, connecting stalk, intraembryonic and yolk sac vessels then join to complete a single vascular system, and primitive blood cells from the yolk sac spread throughout it. An effective means of transport between the villi of the placenta and the embryonic tissues is thus established, and the fluid within it contains primitive red blood cells specialized for the transport of oxygen. Cells from the yolk sac also settle in other sites where blood formation later occurs.

Within the embryo, the blood vessels of each side meet in the wall of the pericardial cavity and form the heart tube which pumps blood around the circulation. Blood returns to the heart via the *cardinal* (intraembryonic), *umbilical* (from the placenta via the connecting stalk) and *vitelline* (yolk sac) *veins*. From the heart, blood passes via *aortic arches* into the *aortae* which give off *intersegmental* (passing between somites), *vitelline* and *umbilical* arteries.

In an animal such as the shark, the heart receives deoxygenated blood from the tissues and delivers it, via symmetrical aortic arches, to the gills whence blood vessels deliver oxygenated blood directly to the tissues. In mammals, however, the heart is partitioned in such a way that its right side receives deoxygenated blood from the tissues and delivers it to the lungs whereas its left side receives oxygenated blood from the lungs and delivers it to the tissues. Although a single organ, the mammalian heart consists of twin pumps placed in series between the pulmonary and the systemic circulations.

In the fetus the lungs are unexpanded and blood flow through them is limited because oxygenation occurs in the placenta. Nevertheless, the left side of the heart must be prepared to assume its full load after birth. The fetal circulation is thus balanced by two right-to-left shunts: one—the *foramen ovale*—from the right atrium to the left atrium, and the other—the *ductus arteriosus*—between a pulmonary artery and the aorta.

After birth the blood flow through the lungs increases as they inflate, circulation through the placenta ceases and the foramen ovale and ductus arteriosus are closed.

Early Vascular System and Gills, Lungs or Placenta

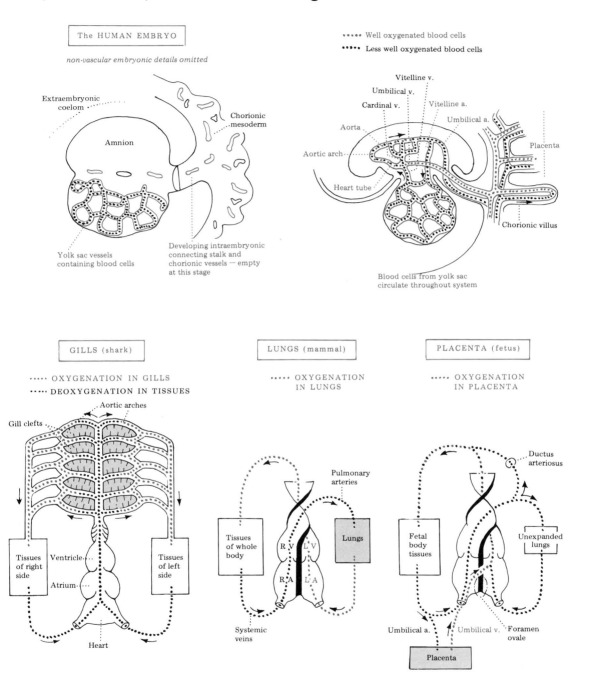

The HUMAN EMBRYO

non-vascular embryonic details omitted

Well oxygenated blood cells

Less well oxygenated blood cells

Extraembryonic coelom

Chorionic mesoderm

Amnion

Yolk sac vessels containing blood cells

Developing intraembryonic connecting stalk and chorionic vessels — empty at this stage

Vitelline v.

Umbilical v.

Cardinal v.

Vitelline a.

Aorta

Umbilical a.

Aortic arch

Placenta

Heart tube

Chorionic villus

Blood cells from yolk sac circulate throughout system

GILLS (shark)

OXYGENATION IN GILLS

DEOXYGENATION IN TISSUES

Aortic arches

Gill clefts

Tissues of right side

Ventricle

Atrium

Tissues of left side

Heart

LUNGS (mammal)

OXYGENATION IN LUNGS

Pulmonary arteries

Tissues of whole body

R V L V

R A L A

Lungs

Systemic veins

PLACENTA (fetus)

OXYGENATION IN PLACENTA

Ductus arteriosus

Fetal body tissues

Unexpanded lungs

Umbilical a.

Umbilical v.

Foramen ovale

Placenta

Blood formation

In the yolk sac wall certain mesenchyme cells form primitive blood vessels. Others within them differentiate into *colony-forming units* (CFUs) which are the stem cells for blood cells of all types. The CFUs undergo proliferative and quantal mitoses, the first clones accumulating haemoglobin and entering the large-celled primitive erythrocyte series. This is superseded by the smaller-celled definitive erythrocyte series. Circulating red cells of both series are at first nucleated and contain only fetal haemoglobin (Hb-F), which takes up oxygen and gives up carbon dioxide more readily than does adult haemoglobin (Hb-A). However, at term, erythrocytes contain about four times as much Hb-F as Hb-A. In subsequent genera-

tions the proportion falls rapidly.

Other cell types appear in sequence and CFUs seed a succession of other sites, where they produce clones. Some CFUs remain pluripotent but others become the progenitors of a progressively more limited range of cell types. In particular, cells seeding the thymus become the progenitors of T lymphocytes. The progenitors of other cell types, including B lymphocytes, are initially found at each of the other sites but later become limited to the bone marrow.

Progenitor cells are not sufficiently differentiated to be recognized by microscopy but can be distinguished by the regulatory factors (glycoproteins) to which they respond and the clones they produce. All bone marrow is of the red haemopoietic type throughout infancy and early childhood.

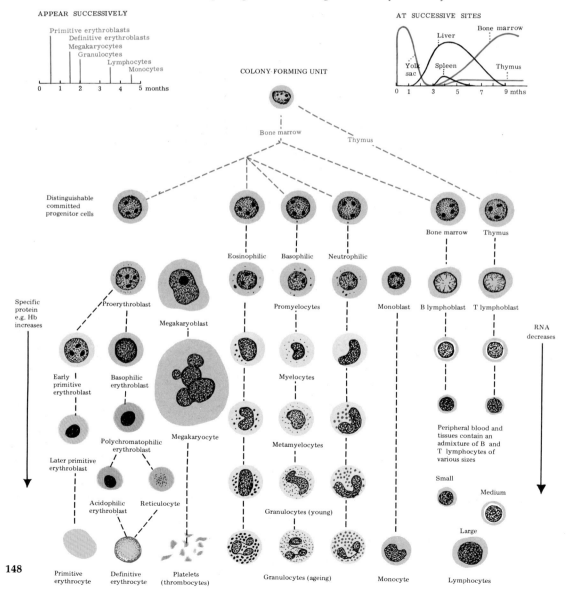

APPEAR SUCCESSIVELY

Primitive erythroblasts
Definitive erythroblasts
Megakaryocytes
Granulocytes
Lymphocytes
Monocytes

0 1 2 3 4 5 months

AT SUCCESSIVE SITES

Bone marrow
Liver
Yolk sac
Spleen
Thymus

0 1 3 5 7 9 mths

COLONY-FORMING UNIT

Bone marrow   Thymus

Distinguishable committed progenitor cells

Eosinophilic   Basophilic   Neutrophilic

Bone marrow   Thymus

Specific protein e.g. Hb increases

Proerythroblast

Promyelocytes

Monoblast   B lymphoblast   T lymphoblast

RNA decreases

Megakaryoblast

Early primitive erythroblast

Basophilic erythroblast

Myelocytes

Polychromatophilic erythroblast

Megakaryocyte

Peripheral blood and tissues contain an admixture of B and T lymphocytes of various sizes

Later primitive erythroblast

Metamyelocytes

Small

Medium

Acidophilic erythroblast   Reticulocyte

Large

Granulocytes (young)

Primitive erythrocyte   Definitive erythrocyte   Platelets (thrombocytes)   Granulocytes (ageing)   Monocyte   Lymphocyte

148

The early circulation

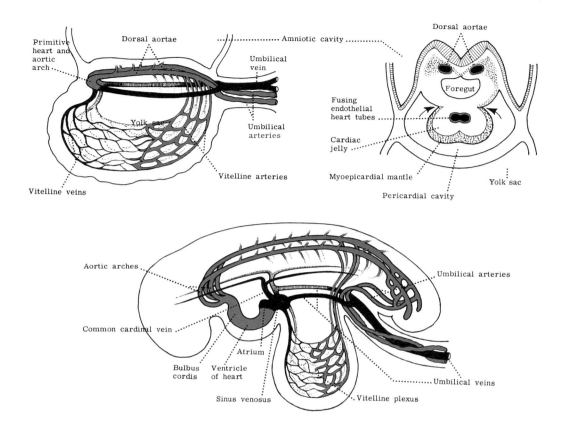

Primitive heart and aortic arch · · ·
Dorsal aortae
Amniotic cavity
Umbilical vein
Yolk sac
Umbilical arteries
Vitelline arteries
Vitelline veins

Dorsal aortae
Foregut
Fusing endothelial heart tubes · · ·
Cardiac jelly · · ·
Myoepicardial mantle
Yolk sac
Pericardial cavity

Aortic arches
Common cardinal vein
Bulbus cordis
Ventricle of heart
Sinus venosus
Atrium
Vitelline plexus
Umbilical arteries
Umbilical veins

The earliest blood vessels are simple endothelial tubes which differentiate in situ in the somatopleuric mesoderm of the chorion, the allantoic mesoderm of the connecting stalk, the splanchnopleuric mesoderm of the yolk sac and, somewhat later, in intraembryonic mesenchyme. From these centres, *chorionic, umbilical, vitelline* and *intraembryonic* systems extend by differentiation in situ of further vessels until they join and a primitive, bilaterally symmetrical, circulation is established. Thereafter, new vessels form as outgrowths of existing vessels whenever and wherever there are functional demands. *Diffuse capillary plexuses precede defined channels in any region.* Such channels arise by the enlargement of some vessels at the expense of others in response to genetic and local haemodynamic influences. All vessels are initially endothelial but are named arteries and veins in anticipation of the development of medial and ad-

ventitial coats from surrounding mesenchyme.

Similarly, the *heart* is first represented by a pair of endothelial tubes which differentiate in the cardiogenic area. With head-fold formation the tubes fuse ventral to the foregut and bulge into the primitive pericardial cavity. The cavity extends dorsally and then medially so that the heart is suspended within it by a *dorsal mesocardium*. Outside the endothelial tubes is a loose *gelatinoreticulum*. This is invaded by myoblasts which are derived from the epicardium and, with it, form the *myoepicardial mantle*. Caudal to the fusing heart tubes is the mesoderm of the septum transversum. In it the vitelline, umbilical and intraembryonic—*common cardinal*—veins empty via a short venous trunk—the *sinus venosus*—into the *primitive atrium* of each side. The atria lead to the single *primitive ventricle*. A single *bulbus cordis* then leads to the *aortic arches* and *dorsal aortae*.

149

The heart

Growing within the confined space of the pericardial cavity, the primitive heart tube folds on itself and forms a *bulboventricular loop* which falls to the right, probably under the influence of flow and of ciliary action of the coelomic epithelium. The notch between the two limbs of this loop becomes shallower as the proximal part of the bulbus merges with the primitive ventricle into a common chamber. *Interventricular sulci* soon appear and demarcate the definitive right and left ventricles. Meanwhile, the primitive atria merge into a *common atrium* which rises out of the septum transversum into the pericardial cavity to lie dorsal to the ventricles. On each side the sinus venosus also rises to lie dorsal to the atrium.

At first the *sinuatrial junction* is ill-defined, but it soon becomes invaginated on each side. Of the resulting folds, that on the left is more extensive and forms a septum which displaces the sinuatrial orifice to the right, creating a transverse chamber—the *body of the sinus venosus*—connecting the two sides (*horns*). The free edges of the folds are now termed *venous valves*.

Meanwhile, the left vitelline and left and right umbilical veins have lost their connections with the sinus venosus (p. 156) and an evagination—the future *common pulmonary vein*—has grown from the sinuatrial junction into the dorsal mesocardium and has tapped the pulmonary venous plexus. The terminal part of the right vitelline vein now connects the liver and the right horn of the sinus venosus and is called the *right hepatocardiac vein*. The common pulmonary vein, and hence the pulmonary venous return, is now relegated to the left atrium as the sinuatrial septum has grown across caudal to it and the interatrial septum primum has appeared on its right.

The *septum primum* is a sickle-shaped projection, produced by proliferation of myoblasts, which grows down towards the narrowing atrioventricular junction in which persisting gelatinoreticulum forms *endocardial cushions*. At first these translate the contractions of the myocardium to the endocardial heart and form a primitive valve mechanism. Later, they meet and fuse and separate *left and right atrioventricular canals*. The advancing septum primum and fused cushions bound a narrowing *ostium primum*. This permits the right-to-left shunt which is necessary for the normal development of the left side of the heart. The ostium primum eventually closes but the shunt is maintained because the cranial part of the septum primum breaks down and an *ostium secundum* is formed.

The bloodstream within the bulboventricular loop is directed first caudally, then to the right and then cranially. Where the stream impinges on the wall and is reflected and changes direction, loops and strands grow in from the myoepicardial mantle and interdigitate with outpouchings from the endocardium to form the trabeculae of the ventricles. The ventricles enlarge by deepening on either side of a zone of stasis, which thus forms the *ventricular septum* and the interventricular sulci. The horns of the crescentic septum reach the corresponding atrioventricular cushions.

As the bulboventricular notch shallows, the right side of the atrioventricular canal comes to lie dorsal to the bulbar orifice. At this stage the ostium primum, atrioventricular canal and interventricular foramen form a continuous hiatus between the right and left sides of the heart. After the atrioventricular cushions have fused, the stream from the left atrioventricular canal enters the left ventricle and is ejected via the interventricular foramen into the dorsal part of the bulbar orifice. The right ventricular outflow passes into the ventral part of the bulbar orifice.

The intersection of left dorsal and right ventral streams produces clockwise spiralling as the two streams traverse the bulbus cordis and a short arterial trunk—the *truncus arteriosus*—to reach the origin of the aortic arches—the *aortic sac*. Beginning between the fourth and sixth aortic arches, an *aorticopulmonary septum* grows back between the spiralling streams. In the truncus arteriosus it spirals through 180° so that the aortic channel which is ventral in the sac is dorsal at the bulbotruncal junction—the site of semilunar valve formation.

The bulbus cordis is lined with deformable *cushion tissue* which is pressed aside by the spiralling streams and fills in between them as *bulbar ridges*: they begin at the bulbotruncal junction where they are continuous with the aorticopulmonary septum and lie left and right; traced back in the bulbus they rotate through 90° and end at the ventral and dorsal horns of the ventricular septum respectively. The *right bulbar ridge* reaches the dorsal horn of the ventricular septum by crossing the fused atrioventricular cushions.

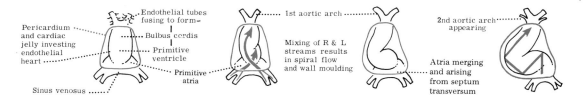

Pericardium and cardiac jelly investing endothelial heart

Endothelial tubes fusing to form

Bulbus cordis

Primitive ventricle

Primitive atria

Sinus venosus

1st aortic arch

Mixing of R & L streams results in spiral flow and wall moulding

2nd aortic arch appearing

Atria merging and arising from septum transversum

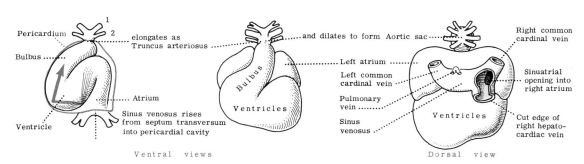

Pericardium

Bulbus

Ventricle

elongates as Truncus arteriosus

Atrium

Sinus venosus rises from septum transversum into pericardial cavity

Bulbus

Ventricles

and dilates to form Aortic sac

Left atrium

Left common cardinal vein

Pulmonary vein

Sinus venosus

Ventricles

Right common cardinal vein

Sinuatrial opening into right atrium

Cut edge of right hepato-cardiac vein

Ventral views

Dorsal view

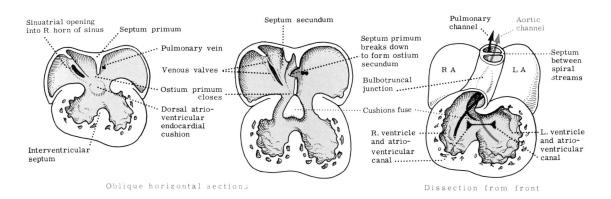

Sinuatrial opening into R. horn of sinus

Septum primum

Pulmonary vein

Venous valves

Ostium primum closes

Dorsal atrio-ventricular endocardial cushion

Interventricular septum

Septum secundum

Septum primum breaks down to form ostium secundum

Bulbotruncal junction

Cushions fuse

R. ventricle and atrio-ventricular canal

Pulmonary channel

Aortic channel

RA

LA

Septum between spiral streams

L. ventricle and atrioventricular canal

Oblique horizontal sections

Dissection from front

BULBOVENTRICULAR & AORTICOPULMONARY SEPTATION

Sections of bulbotruncal junction

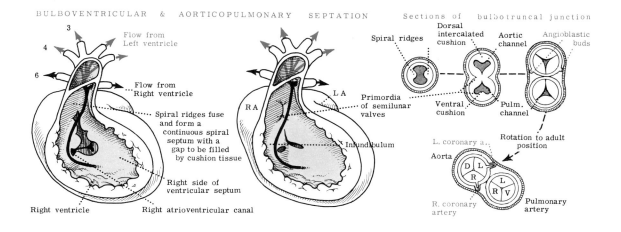

3

4

6

Flow from Left ventricle

Flow from Right ventricle

Spiral ridges fuse and form a continuous spiral septum with a gap to be filled by cushion tissue

Right side of ventricular septum

Right ventricle

Right atrioventricular canal

RA

LA

Infundibulum

Spiral ridges

Dorsal intercalated cushion

Aortic channel

Angioblastic buds

Primordia of semilunar valves

Ventral cushion

Pulm. channel

Rotation to adult position

L. coronary a.

Aorta

R. coronary artery

D | L
R

L | V
R

Pulmonary artery

Beginning at the bulbotruncal junction, the bulbar ridges meet, fuse and are reinforced by the ingrowth of muscle tissue. The resulting septum divides the bulbus into a major part—the *infundibulum* of the right ventricle—and a minor part—the *aortic vestibule*. The remaining gap between the bulbar septum and the ventricular septum is closed by cushion tissue from the right side of the fused atrioventricular cushions. This grows along the crest of the ventricular septum, fusing with it and the bulbar septum, and eventually forms the *membranous part of the interventricular septum*. At the bulbotruncal junction, bisected *right and left septal cushions*, with an additional (*nonseptal*) cushion in each channel, form the primordia of the semilunar valves. Flow conditions produce excavation of their downstream aspects to form cusps and sinuses.

The bulbar septum separates the *outflow tract of the right ventricle*—the infundibulum—from the *outflow tract of the left ventricle*—the aortic vestibule. The outflow tracts lie ventral to the atrioventricular canals, which have accumulations of cushion tissue projecting into them. In the *left canal, septal and lateral cushions* are the primordia of the anterior and posterior leaflets of the mitral valve. In the *right canal*, there is a single *septal cushion*—the primordium of the septal leaflet of the tricuspid valve—but there are two *lateral cushions*. These are derived largely from the right bulbar ridge and are the primordia of the anterior and posterior leaflets. The shafts of muscle trabeculae which extend into the bases of the cushions, split off from the ventricular wall, while the cushions themselves become excavated on their downstream aspects to form valve cusps. The mural ends of the trabeculae remain muscular and form papillary muscles. Collagen fibres are deposited in their cushion ends which form the chordae tendineae attached to the valve cusps.

Meanwhile, a sickle-shaped *septum secundum* grows down from the atrial roof and obtrudes on the ostium secundum. The part of the septum primum attached to the endocardial cushions becomes a flap slung from the left side of the septum secundum. The resulting *atrial septal complex* consists of a *foramen ovale* bounded by a *limbus* (septum secundum) and a flap-like *valve* (septum primum). It is a competent valve system which permits a right-to-left shunt but prevents a left-to-right shunt. The common pulmonary vein and its right and left tributaries have dilated and have been incorporated into the *left atrium* as the smooth-walled vestibule. The primitive left atrium with its ridged lining is represented only by the auricular appendage. The right horn of the sinus venosus has also dilated and has been incorporated into the *right atrium* as the smooth-walled sinus venarum. The vessels which formerly opened into the right horn now drain directly into this part of the right atrium. These vessels are the right common cardinal vein, the right hepatocardiac vein and the body of the sinus venosus. They form the proximal parts of the superior vena cava, the inferior vena cava and the coronary sinus respectively. The intermediate part of the coronary sinus is derived from the left horn of the sinus venosus, and the distal part from the left common cardinal vein. The venous valves, which formerly bounded the sinuatrial opening, are now much reduced. The left venous valve fuses with the atrial septal complex. The right venous valve, though reduced by resorption, continues to separate the ridged primitive right atrium from the derivatives of the sinus venosus and forms the crista terminalis, most of the valve of the inferior vena cava and the valve of the coronary sinus. The valve of the inferior vena cava is completed by the spur of tissue which separates the orifices of the inferior vena cava and coronary sinus.

The cardiac myoblasts form a non-syncytial network. They develop myofibrils which increase in number and size, align with those of adjoining cells and develop cross-striations. At first atrial and ventricular myocardium are continuous across the atrioventricular junction. The *atrioventricular bundle* is then seen as a specialized fascicle with densely staining nuclei which extends from the right side of the dorsal wall of the common atrium, behind the dorsal atrioventricular cushion, on to the crest of the primitive ventricular septum. Later, the atrioventricular node is defined at its atrial end, and left and right branches appear successively at its ventricular end. Elsewhere, continuity across the atrioventricular junction is lost as the fibrous skeleton of the heart develops. The sinuatrial node develops in relation to the base of the right venous valve.

Interatrial and Atrioventricular Valve Formation

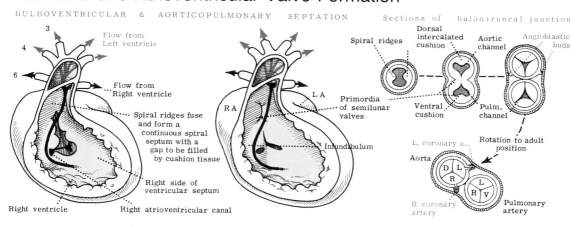

3

4

6

Flow from Left ventricle

Flow from Right ventricle

Spiral ridges fuse and form a continuous spiral septum with a gap to be filled by cushion tissue

Right side of ventricular septum

Right ventricle

Right atrioventricular canal

R A

L A

Infundibulum

Spiral ridges

Dorsal intercalated cushion

Aortic channel

Angioblastic buds

Ventral cushion

Pulm. channel

Primordia of semilunar valves

Rotation to adult position

L. coronary a.

Aorta

D L
R

L
R V

R. coronary artery

Pulmonary artery

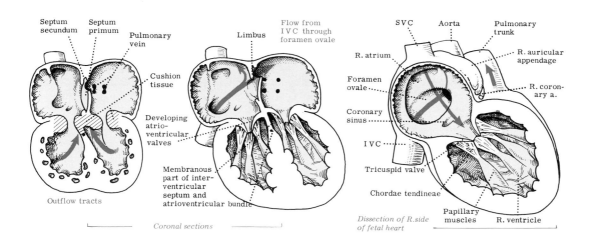

Septum secundum

Septum primum

Pulmonary vein

Cushion tissue

Developing atrioventricular valves

Membranous part of interventricular septum and atrioventricular bundle

Outflow tracts

Limbus

Flow from IVC through foramen ovale

Coronal sections

SVC

Aorta

Pulmonary trunk

R. atrium

R. auricular appendage

Foramen ovale

R. coronary a.

Coronary sinus

IVC

Tricuspid valve

Chordae tendineae

Papillary muscles

R. ventricle

Dissection of R. side of fetal heart

The Pericardium

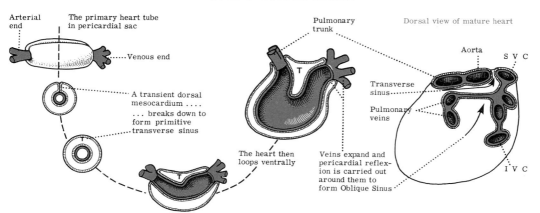

Arterial end

The primary heart tube in pericardial sac

Venous end

A transient dorsal mesocardium ....
... breaks down to form primitive transverse sinus

The heart then loops ventrally

Veins expand and pericardial reflexion is carried out around them to form Oblique Sinus

Dorsal view of mature heart

Pulmonary trunk

Aorta

SVC

Transverse sinus

Pulmonary veins

IVC

The arteries

The *aortic arch arteries* appear in the mesenchyme of the pharyngeal arches in craniocaudal sequence and connect the *aortic sac* with the two *dorsal aortae*. These fuse between the fourth lumbar and fourth thoracic segments and form the single descending aorta. As new arches appear, the flow pattern within the system changes and blood is diverted from preceding arches. The first two arches thus become redundant and do not persist as complete arches. With the development of the neck and descent of the heart from its primitive cervical position, the third and fourth arches draw out the aortic sac on each side to form *right* and *left horns*. The part related to the third arch further elongates and forms the common carotid artery. From this the external carotid artery sprouts as a new formation, though it may incorporate segments of the first two arches. The proximal part of the internal carotid artery is derived from the third arch itself. The distal part is derived from cranial extensions of the dorsal aorta, including segments of the first two arches. The fourth arches persist as channels connecting the horns of the aortic sac, via the corresponding dorsal aorta, to the upper limb artery. The right horn thus forms the brachiocephalic trunk, and the right fourth arch the proximal part of the subclavian artery. The aortic sac and its left horn and fourth arch form the arch of the aorta. The fifth pair of arches is transient or absent in man.

The sixth arches are atypical. They supply primitive pulmonary plexuses and only secondarily become connected with the dorsal aortae. The ventral stems become the pulmonary arteries. On the right side connection with the dorsal aorta is lost, but on the left it persists as the *ductus arteriosus*. The dorsal aortae between the third and fourth arches and the unfused part of the right dorsal aorta distal to the limb artery then disappear. Meanwhile, the spiral ridges have fused and separated the pulmonary trunk (leading from the right ventricle to sixth arch derivatives) from the ascending aorta (leading via the arch of the aorta and the brachiocephalic trunk to fourth arch derivatives).

Specialized pressor-receptor areas (e.g. carotid sinus) develop in persisting arches and are supplied by the appropriate arch nerves. The recurrent laryngeal nerves reach the larynx by passing caudal to the sixth arch on each side. On the left, this arch (ductus arteriosus) descends into the thorax, dragging a loop of nerve with it. On the right, the sixth arch loses connection with the dorsal aorta, and the fifth is transient so the nerve slips these arches and hooks around the fourth arch (subclavian artery), thus descending only to the root of the neck.

The primitive dorsal aortae lead directly to the umbilical arteries and develop, in turn, ventral segmental (vitelline) branches, dorsolateral intersegmental (somatic) branches, lateral segmental (intermediate) branches and longitudinal anastomoses which connect the different levels. The caudal loops of the umbilical arteries are bypassed by anastomotic connections with the fifth lumbar intersegmental arteries which pass dorsal and lateral to the Wolffian duct. The paired *ventral segmental branches* fuse and are reduced to the midline arteries of the foregut (oesophageal and coeliac trunk), midgut (superior mesenteric) and hindgut (inferior mesenteric). Dorsal splanchnic anastomoses form the gastroepiploic and pancreaticoduodenal arteries and the mesenteric arcades. Ventral anastomoses form the gastric and hepatic arteries. The *dorsolateral intersegmental branches* form the posterior intercostal, subcostal and lumbar arteries and the stems of the limb arteries. The *longitudinal somatic anastomoses* and their derivatives are post-transverse (deep cervical), postcostal (most of the vertebral), prelaminar and postcentral (spinal), precostal (ascending cervical; supreme intercostal) and ventral (internal thoracic; superior and inferior epigastric). The *lateral segmental branches* form the phrenic, suprarenal, renal and gonadal arteries.

The developing *brain* is covered by a capillary plexus fed by the branches of the internal carotid artery. Its primitive maxillary branch supplies the telencephalon but is succeeded by a terminal branch which gives rise to the anterior and middle cerebral and choroidal arteries. The diencephalon and mesencephalon are supplied by another terminal branch which gives rise to the posterior communicating and cerebral and the anterior cerebellar arteries. The arteries of the hindbrain and cord differentiate from longitudinal plexuses fed by presegmental branches of the internal carotid artery and by spinal branches of intersegmental arteries. On each side the capillary plexuses drain into the precardinal vein (p. 156) via a *primary head vein*: this lies medial to the trigeminal ganglion, where it persists as the cavernous sinus. Secondary connections between the plexuses develop dorsal to the primary head veins and supersede them as main channels. The deeper vessels form the cerebral veins whilst the more superficial vessels form dural venous sinuses.

The Aortic Arches

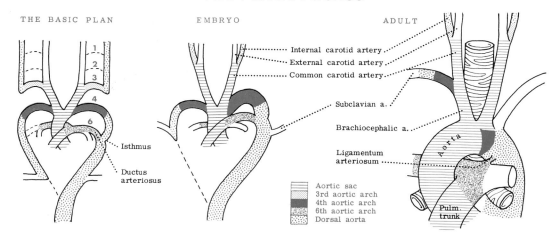

Internal carotid artery
External carotid artery
Common carotid artery

Subclavian a.

Brachiocephalic a.

Ligamentum arteriosum

Isthmus

Ductus arteriosus

Aorta

Pulm. trunk

Aortic sac
3rd aortic arch
4th aortic arch
6th aortic arch
Dorsal aorta

Segmental Arteries and Longitudinal Anastomoses

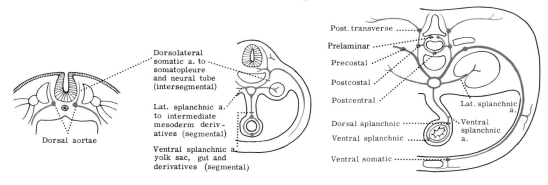

Dorsolateral somatic a. to somatopleure and neural tube (intersegmental)

Lat. splanchnic a. to intermediate mesoderm derivatives (segmental)

Ventral splanchnic a. yolk sac, gut and derivatives (segmental)

Dorsal aortae

Post. transverse
Prelaminar
Precostal
Postcostal
Postcentral
Dorsal splanchnic
Ventral splanchnic
Ventral somatic

Lat. splanchnic a.
Ventral splanchnic a.

Dural Venous Sinuses

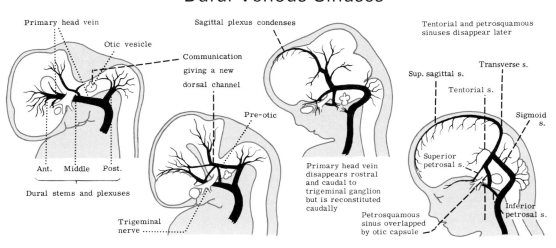

Primary head vein

Otic vesicle

Sagittal plexus condenses

Communication giving a new dorsal channel

Tentorial and petrosquamous sinuses disappear later

Transverse s.

Sup. sagittal s.

Tentorial s.

Sigmoid s.

Superior petrosal s.

Pre-otic

Ant. Middle Post.

Dural stems and plexuses

Primary head vein disappears rostral and caudal to trigeminal ganglion but is reconstituted caudally

Inferior petrosal s.

Trigeminal nerve

Petrosquamous sinus overlapped by otic capsule

155

The veins and lymphatics

The intrinsic veins of the somite embryo are the *precardinal* and *postcardinal* veins which join to form a *common cardinal vein* on each side.

The right *precardinal vein* forms the right internal jugular and brachiocephalic veins and that part of the superior vena cava cranial to the azygos vein. Caudal to the azygos vein the superior vena cava is derived from the right common cardinal vein. An oblique cross-connection between the precardinal veins forms part of the left brachiocephalic vein. As venous return is thus diverted to the right, the left common cardinal vein retrogresses and forms the distal part of the coronary sinus, the oblique vein of the left atrium and a fibrous connection between it and the proximal parts of the left pre- and postcardinal veins. These parts form the left superior intercostal vein which drains upwards into the left brachiocephalic vein. The left precardinal vein forms the rest of the left brachiocephalic vein and the left internal jugular vein.

The *postcardinal veins* drain the lower limb buds, the body wall and the mesonephric ridge and lie dorsolateral to the last-named. They are soon supplemented and largely superseded by other longitudinal channels and plexiform connections. The venous drainage of the mesonephric ridges is taken over by *subcardinal veins* lying medial to them and ventral to the aorta. That of the body wall is taken over by *supracardinal* and *azygos line veins* which lie dorsal to the aorta and lateral and medial to the sympathetic trunk. With the diversion of venous return to the right, most of the channels on the left disappear. Those that persist drain to the right by cross-anastomoses. Beginning caudally, the inferior vena cava is formed from the right postcardinal vein (draining lower limb and pelvis), the right supracardinal vein (draining lower abdominal wall), the right subcardinal vein (draining kidneys, suprarenals and gonads), the right hepatocardiac vein (representing hepatic sinusoids and the terminal part of the right vitelline vein draining the liver) and anastomotic segments between them.

The further development of the *visceral veins* is linked with that of the liver. As the vitelline veins pass cranially, a *dorsal* and two *ventral anastomoses* connect them and form a figure 8 around the primitive duodenum. Beyond this they break up into hepatic sinusoids. Their cranial ends still drain into the sinus venosus as hepatocardiac veins and are connected by a *subdiaphragmatic anastomosis*. A midline channel—the *ductus venosus*—connects the subdiaphragmatic and the cranial duodenal anastomoses. With expansion of the liver and diversion of venous return to the right side of the heart, the right umbilical and left hepatocardiac veins disappear completely and the left umbilical vein, after being tapped by the liver sinusoids and cranial duodenal anastomosis, disappears in its cranial part. The whole of the placental venous return then traverses the liver, but whereas some traverses the sinusoids, the rest traverses the ductus venosus which effectively connects the left umbilical and right hepatocardiac veins.

Parts of the vitelline veins also disappear in such a way that the persisting parts of the figure 8 system may be represented as a letter S. However, since the developing duodenum is meanwhile assuming its characteristic C shape, the persisting parts pursue a progressively straighter course to the liver. The superior mesenteric vein and, later, the splenic vein join the left end of the original dorsal anastomosis which thus, with the extrahepatic part of the right vitelline vein, forms the portal vein. The more distal parts of the vitelline system disappear with the vitellointestinal duct.

The earliest *lymph vessels* may be derived from clefts in mesenchyme which become secondarily connected with the venous system, or they may be derived directly by capillary offshoots from the venous system. They form a bilaterally symmetrical system with transverse anastomoses across the midline. Some confluesce and form lymph sacs. Paired sacs are found in relation to the veins at the roots of the limbs, and midline sacs in the root of the mesentery. New lymph vessels bud off from the sacs or arises in situ and connect with them. The lymph sacs at the roots of the upper limbs have, or develop, connection with the internal jugular veins and, via bilateral anastomotic connections with the midline sacs, form bilateral primitive thoracic ducts. The definitive thoracic duct is derived from the caudal part of the right vessel, a transverse anastomosis and the cranial part of the left vessel. The right lymphatic duct is derived from the cranial part of the right vessel. The lymph sacs mainly retrogress but a midline sac persists as the cisterna chyli. Mesenchyme aggregates around the others and around more peripheral lymphatics, and is seeded by lymphocytes to form lymph nodes.

The Somatic Veins

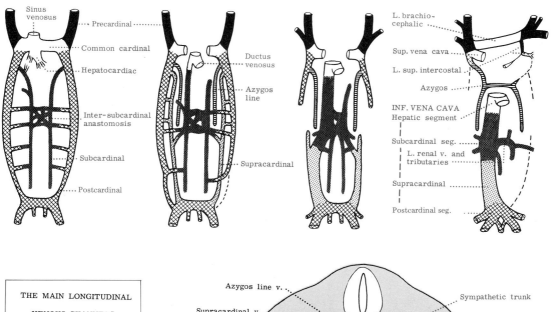

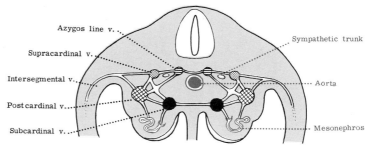

THE MAIN LONGITUDINAL
VENOUS CHANNELS
OF THE TRUNK
AND THEIR ANASTOMOTIC
CONNECTIONS

The Visceral Veins

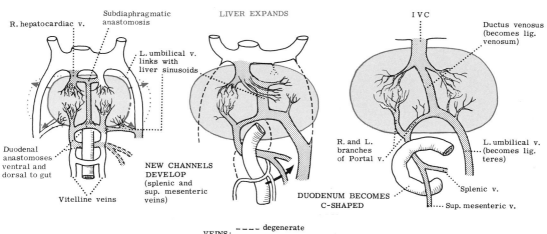

VEINS: – – – – degenerate
░░░░ persist

Fetal and neonatal circulation

Cardiovascular development before birth has led to a system which is adequate for prenatal needs and yet capable of undergoing changes at birth which fit it for postnatal needs. Fairly well-oxygenated blood returns from the placenta via the unpaired vein in the umbilical cord and via the persisting left umbilical vein in the body. Some of this blood discharges into hepatic sinusoids but the rest bypasses them, is joined by blood from the portal vein and traverses the ductus venosus. It is then joined by blood from the hepatic veins and prehepatic inferior vena cava. The inferior vena caval blood is directed forwards and to the left, and the stream is divided by the limbus of the foramen ovale—*crista dividens*—into left atrial and right atrial streams. Perhaps some three-quarters of the inferior caval stream passes through the *foramen ovale* into the left atrium, where it is joined by blood from the pulmonary veins. The mixture passes into the left ventricle and is ejected into the aorta, whence most of this *relatively well-oxygenated blood reaches the arteries of the heart, head, neck and arms.* The residuum traverses the *isthmus aortae* to join the stream from the *ductus arteriosus.* Meanwhile, the remainder of the inferior caval stream joins the blood from the superior vena cava and coronary sinus in the right atrium proper and enters the right ventricle. Some of the right ventricular blood goes to the lungs. The remainder bypasses them via the ductus arteriosus and joins the stream from the isthmus aortae in the descending aorta for distribution partly to the lower parts of the body but mainly via the umbilical arteries to the placenta.

Both ventricles are thus working in parallel, and at birth their walls are of similar thickness. However, because they work in parallel, their outputs need not be, and probably are not, equal. Similarly, the placenta and lungs are in parallel with the systemic body tissues. The placenta constitutes a relatively low-resistance circuit and has a greater volume of blood flow than the systemic tissues. The unexpanded fetal lungs constitute a relatively high-resistance circuit and have a smaller volume of blood flow than the systemic tissues.

At term, the principal cardiovascular and respiratory reflexes are believed to be active. During delivery the oxygen saturation in the umbilical arteries falls below 30 per cent. This is probably due to compression of the umbilical cord, to partial separation of the placenta and to a reduction in uterine blood flow during contractions. Respiration is then stimulated reflexly by the effect of anoxia on chemoreceptors, and probably by exteroceptive stimuli. With the onset of respiration, intrathoracic pressure falls and the lungs are inflated. Pulmonary vascular resistance falls rapidly and the pulmonary blood flow increases up to tenfold in as many minutes. This response is partly due to gaseous expansion of the lungs, a local mechanical phenomenon, and partly due to changes in alveolar and arterial oxygen and carbon dioxide tensions.

As the blood flow increases, the pulmonary arterial pressure falls and the left atrial pressure rises. Furthermore, when the venous return from the placenta ceases, the inferior vena caval pressure falls. These circumstances combine to press the valve of the foramen ovale against the limbus and produce *functional closure.* As this functional closure depends on relative pressures on the two sides of the valve, there may be an intermittent flow of blood from the inferior vena cava into the left atrium for some days after birth. Left atrial pressure, however, continues to rise, the shunt ceases and the valve begins to fuse with the limbus. During the following months the connective tissue of the valve increases, and structural closure usually occurs, forming the *fossa ovalis.*

The muscular wall of the *ductus arteriosus* contracts within a few minutes of birth, due to the direct action of oxygen or of catecholamines. For up to an hour the reduced shunt continues to be right-to-left in the fetal direction, but after this time the increase in systemic arterial pressure and the decrease in pulmonary arterial pressure combine to reverse the shunt, which may then produce a characteristic innocent heart murmur. These pressure changes are associated with a rapid adjustment of ventricular preponderance. This occurs mainly in the first month, as the right ventricle atrophies and the left ventricle hypertrophies. The degree of left ventricular preponderance characteristic of later life is reached by 6 months. Some days after birth (longer in premature infants) the ductus arteriosus shuts down completely. It becomes occluded by overgrowth of the intima and media, subsequently undergoing fibrosis and contraction to form the *ligamentum arteriosum.* The umbilical arteries contract early, and before the umbilical vein and ductus venosus, so an appreciable amount of fetal blood is able to return from the placenta if the umbilical cord is not clamped immediately. Closure of the placental low-resistance circuit leads to a rise in systemic vascular resistance. The vessels ultimately become obliterated, forming the obliterated umbilical arteries, the ligamentum teres (umbilical vein) and the ligamentum venosum (ductus venosus).

Fetal Circulation

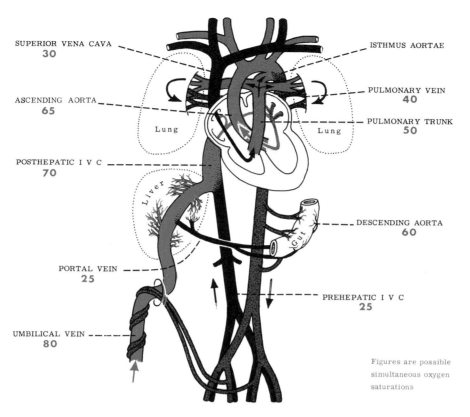

SUPERIOR VENA CAVA
30

ASCENDING AORTA
65

POSTHEPATIC I V C
70

PORTAL VEIN
25

UMBILICAL VEIN
80

ISTHMUS AORTAE

PULMONARY VEIN
40

PULMONARY TRUNK
50

DESCENDING AORTA
60

PREHEPATIC I V C
25

Lung

Lung

Liver

Gut

Figures are possible
simultaneous oxygen
saturations

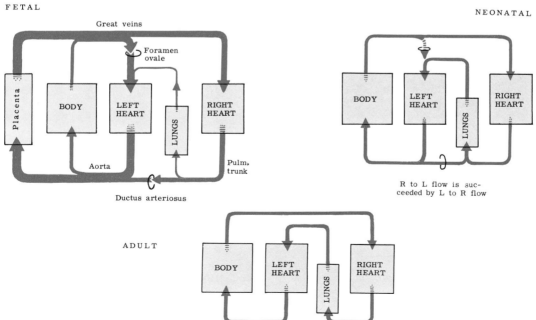

FETAL

Great veins

Foramen ovale

Placenta

BODY

LEFT HEART

LUNGS

RIGHT HEART

Aorta

Pulm. trunk

Ductus arteriosus

NEONATAL

BODY

LEFT HEART

LUNGS

RIGHT HEART

R to L flow is suc-
ceeded by L to R flow

ADULT

BODY

LEFT HEART

LUNGS

RIGHT HEART

Anomalies

As a group, malformations of the heart are the commonest serious congenital conditions and have an incidence of about 6 per 1000 total births. Of these, about 20 per cent each have a ventricular septal defect or a persistent ductus arteriosus; about 10 per cent each have an atrial septal defect, isolated pulmonary stenosis, Fallot's tetralogy or transposition of the arterial trunks or coarctation of the aorta while 10 per cent have other less common malformations of which more than a hundred varieties have been described.

In its commonest form an *isolated ventricular septal defect* occurs at the site of the membranous part of the interventricular septum and thus represents the failure of cushion tissue to bridge the gap between the bulbar and ventricular septa. In this case the atrioventricular bundle lies in the free edge of the septum and is vulnerable during surgical repair. Much less commonly the defect is in the muscular part of the interventricular septum and represents excessive outpouching and breakdown of the endocardium between trabeculae. In this case the defect may close spontaneously. In either form there is a left-to-right shunt between the ventricles.

Failure of the processes of muscular contraction and intimal proliferation which normally close it, results in a *persistent ductus arteriosus* and in persistence of the left-to-right shunt of neonatal life. Spontaneous closure may eventually occur but ligation in childhood, not only to close the shunt but also to reduce the risk of infective endarteritis, is preferred.

By far the commonest *atrial septal defect* is an *ostium secundum defect* in which the valve is inadequate to cover the foramen ovale or is fenestrated and thus is incompetent and permits a left-to-right shunt. In some normal individuals, structural closure may fail to occur but, provided the valve is competent, this is of no significance. *Endocardial cushion defects* are less common and occur in three degrees. In the first, the septum primum is underdeveloped or fails to fuse with the atrioventricular cushions, resulting in a *persistent ostium primum*. In the second, the atrioventricular cushions fail to fuse with each other, resulting in a *persistent common atrioventricular canal*. In the third, the atrioventricular cushions also fail to fuse with the ventricular septum and result in a *defect of the membranous septum*. Thus in the third degree a continuous hiatus persists between the left and right sides of the heart.

Isolated pulmonary stenosis is commoner than *aortic stenosis* and may affect the pulmonary valve or the infundibulum. It is also common in combination with hypertrophy of the right ventricle and a ventricular septal defect, with the aorta over-riding it, in *Fallot's tetralogy*. This combination produces a right-to-left shunt and central cyanosis—the classic 'blue baby'.

In *transposition of the arterial trunks* the aorticopulmonary septum has failed to spiral, so the aorta arises from the right ventricle and the pulmonary trunk from the left. The condition is incompatible with postnatal life unless accompanied by a bidirectional shunt (through a septal defect or a persistent ductus) or by transposition of the whole or part of the heart so that the arterial transposition is 'corrected' and the connections are appropriate. Less commonly, the aorticopulmonary septum is absent in whole—*persistent truncus arteriosus*—or in part—*aorticopulmonary window*.

In *coarctation of the aorta* (L. *arctare* = to tighten) a constriction is present, usually near the ductus arteriosus, which may persist. Coarctation at this site may represent a persistent isthmus aortae or involvement of the aorta in the closing mechanisms of the ductus. However, coarctation also occurs beyond the ductus and even, rarely, beyond the diaphragm, so other factors must operate. As there is a substantial pressure differential between the two sides of the coarctation, the blood pressure recorded in the upper limbs is higher than in the lower limbs and a collateral circulation develops.

Variations of the aorta other than coarctation are rare. Since flow factors, which can easily vary, are at least in part responsible for determining which blood vessels develop from a network at the expense of others, variations in other blood vessels are common. Similarly, since venous pressure is lower, and thus less determinative, variations in veins are commoner than in arteries. However, in most cases variations are incidental findings and not of pathological significance.

In most cases congenital heart disease is multifactorial. The sex ratio is 1:1 and the incidence in twins is about twice that in non-twins; the incidence in the children and siblings of affected individuals may be 20–30 times higher than in the general population. Mechanical factors may play a part and a whole gamut of anomalies can be produced by deformation of the heart tube. Altitude has effects, and viruses such as rubella may produce persistent ductus arteriosus, stenoses and other lesions.

Rarely, Mendelian inheritance operates. Marfan's syndrome is an autosomal dominant disorder of connective tissue which may be associated with congenital aortic valve disease. Autosomal recessive inheritance operates in *dextrocardia* as part of *situs inversus* (p. 91) and perhaps in some other conditions.

In Down's syndrome (trisomy 21) endocardial cushion defects are common, while with trisomies 13 and 18 ventricular septal defect, persistent ductus arteriosus and other anomalies occur. Aortic stenosis and, less commonly, coarctation of the aorta occur in the monosomic Turner's syndrome (45,X).

VENTRICULAR SEPTAL DEFECT   PERSISTENT DUCTUS ARTERIOSUS   ATRIAL SEPTAL DEFECT

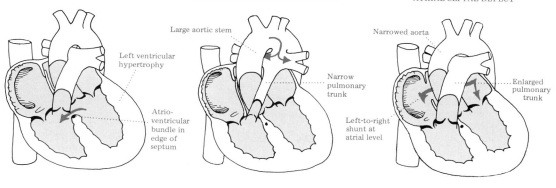

VENTRICULAR SEPTAL DEFECT

Left ventricular
hypertrophy

Atrio-
ventricular
bundle in
edge of
septum

PERSISTENT DUCTUS ARTERIOSUS

Large aortic stem

Narrow
pulmonary
trunk

ATRIAL SEPTAL DEFECT

Narrowed aorta

Enlarged
pulmonary
trunk

Left-to-right
shunt at
atrial level

COMBINED ENDOCARDIAL CUSHION DEFECT   TETRALOGY OF FALLOT   PERSISTENT TRUNCUS ARTERIOSUS

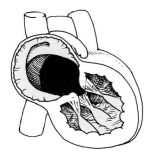

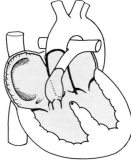

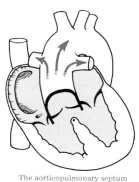

1. Persistent ostium primum
2. Persistent common atrioventricular canal
3. Cleft valve and defect of
   the membranous interventricular septum

1. Pulmonary stenosis
2. Right ventricular hypertrophy
3. Ventricular septal defect
4. Aorta overriding it

The aorticopulmonary septum
is absent and the truncus arises
from both ventricles above a
ventricular septal defect

——— VARIATIONS OF THE AORTA ———

Modified
basic plan

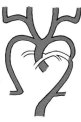

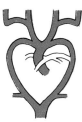

in the
ADULT

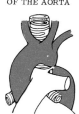

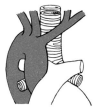

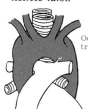

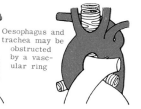

COARCTATION
OF THE AORTA

RIGHT-SIDED
AORTIC ARCH

DOUBLE
AORTIC ARCH

ABERRANT RIGHT
SUBCLAVIAN ARTERY

Oesophagus and
trachea may be
obstructed
by a vasc-
ular ring

161

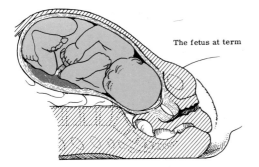

The fetus at term

Cervix dilates

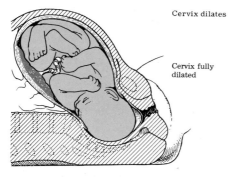

Cervix fully dilated

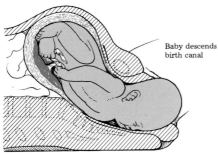

Baby descends birth canal

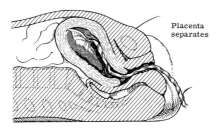

Placenta separates

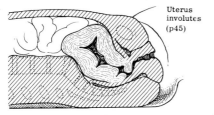

Uterus involutes (p45)

Birth and the Newborn

The fetal period is essentially one of increasing structural and functional maturity. Although the main organ systems are established by the third month, the 8-week fetus is unsuited to extrauterine life in many respects: the nostrils are plugged with epithelium, the palate and nasal septum are unfused and the lungs have bronchioles but no alveoli; the endocrine and exocrine glands are non-functional and the smooth muscle and glands of the hollow viscera have yet to appear; the skeletal muscles are represented but the only elicitable reflex is a mass response to stimulation around the mouth.

By 28 weeks all the basic reflexes are established and the other circumstances detailed have so changed that the fetus may be capable of an independent existence. In some countries the fetus is still pronounced legally *viable* at 28 weeks. In others, the increased chance of survival of younger fetuses has been recognized and a fetus of at least 20 weeks gestation or weighing at least 400 g is legally viable. The termination of pregnancy before legal viability is called an *abortion* or miscarriage, and may be *spontaneous*, *therapeutic* or *criminal*. The termination of pregnancy after legal viability but before 37 weeks is called a *premature labour*.

The early premature baby is lean, red and wrinkled and has abundant lanugo; the head is proportionately large, the eyes are prominent, and the nose is small, flat and, like the ears, contains little cartilage; the tongue seems large; the nails are soft and do not reach the finger tips; the abdomen is protuberant and an umbilical hernia is frequently present; movements are infrequent and sluggish, and cries are feeble. Although *viable*, the infant is notably immature in respect of the respiratory system, temperature regulation, digestive and excretory mechanisms, and in reserves of fat, glycogen, calcium, phosphorus and iron. The respiratory system is immature with respect to lung development itself, to the chemoreceptors which monitor arterial oxygen and carbon dioxide tensions and to the production by the secretory cells of alveoli of the phospholipid surfactant which facilitates the inflation of the lungs. These and other deficiencies are normally made up before delivery at term.

Before the onset of labour the fetal pituitary-adrenal system is activated and fetal cortisol levels rise. This produces not only changes in the fetus (e.g. in synthesis of haemoglobin, thyroxine, glycogen and surfactant) but also in the placenta (enzymes which increase the metabolism of maternal progesterone to oestrogens). As a result, maternal progesterone levels fall and maternal oestrogens induce the synthesis and release of prostaglandin F_{2a} (PGF) by the placenta and uterus and the release of oxytocin by the maternal neurohypophysis. PGF and oxytocin are potent stimulators of uterine activity and initiate labour.

The process of birth or *labour* is considered in three stages, all consequent on active contractions of the uterus. In the *first stage* the cervix uteri dilates to accommodate the fetal head. In the *second stage* the baby descends the birth canal. In the *third stage* the placenta separates and is expelled with the extra-embryonic membranes and decidua. The membranes may rupture early in labour or the child may be born in a caul. The average newborn child weighs some 3500 g, is about 50 cm in length and has head, chest and abdomen circumferences of about 35 cm. The full-term baby is plump and pink and has but little lanugo; the nails have grown beyond the tips of the digits; the breasts of both sexes are enlarged and may secrete *witch's milk*, due to the stimulus of maternal hormones; movements are active and sustained, and cries are lusty.

The vault of the skull has areas of residual membrane called *fontanelles*. These have permitted *moulding* of the fetal head as it adapts to the shape and size of the maternal pelvis in the birth process. Moulding commonly entails the parietals over-riding the occipital bone and each other, and persists in diminishing degree for some days after birth. The middle-ear apparatus is of adult size in infancy and, with the facial nerve, is in some danger as the mastoid process and the bony external acoustic meatus are undeveloped. The maxillary sinus is rudimentary and the face is small but it is broadened by the presence of an encapsulated fat depot in the cheeks, the so-called

sucking pad (p. 166). The tongue is blunt and flat and, lacking the mobile pointed tip of the adult, a later development, may appear *tongue-tied*.

Among the viscera, the thymus is relatively enormous and the transverse diameter of the heart is more than half that of the thorax instead of less; the lungs are small, covering less of the heart than in the adult, and alveolar development is incomplete; the liver and suprarenal glands have diminished in relative size over the months, but are still large in relation to other viscera. At this stage the bladder is an abdominal organ and the testes are below the superficial inguinal ring, if not actually within the scrotum. The prepuce normally remains partially adherent and not fully retractile for several months or a year.

The important sensory pathways, the association pathways of the brain stem and spinal cord, and the motor nerves have been myelinating and functional for some months before birth. The long motor paths, however, do not begin to myelinate until term, and the newborn operates as a brain-stem preparation with little cerebral function, motor reactions being essentially reflex. Tendon reflexes, the light reflex, the tonic neck reflex and other reflexes peculiar to the newborn (p. 166) are present but the superficial reflexes are absent. The special sense organs are functional at birth, but hearing is impaired until the middle ear drains of amniotic fluid. The normal infant will pass a dark green stool—*meconium*—and void urine within the first 24 hours.

Some Features of the Newborn

OSSIFICATION

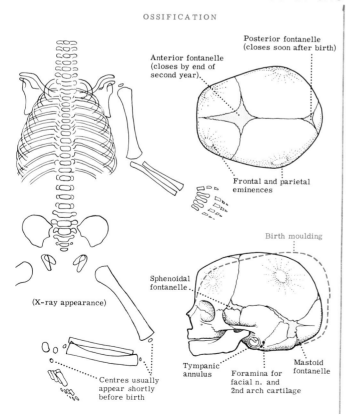

Anterior fontanelle (closes by end of second year)

Posterior fontanelle (closes soon after birth)

Frontal and parietal eminences

Birth moulding

Sphenoidal fontanelle

(X-ray appearance)

Tympanic annulus

Foramina for facial n. and 2nd arch cartilage

Mastoid fontanelle

Centres usually appear shortly before birth

VISCERA

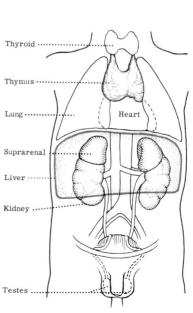

Thyroid

Thymus

Lung

Heart

Suprarenal

Liver

Kidney

Testes

Prenatal and Postnatal Growth

Neither the fetus nor the infant is an adult in miniature. Each has its peculiar features and the transition from the fetus to the adult entails far more than an increase in height and weight. Relatively speaking, the young fetus has an enormous head, practically no neck and small hindquarters. 'The infant is large-headed, short-limbed, squat and rounded, whilst the early adolescent is a slender long-limbed, gazelle-like creature who subsequently is transmuted into the only too familiar sheep-like adult' (Ellis, 1947).

Changes in proportion and size are affected by genetic, hormonal and nutritional factors and occur at

girls with mean durations from 13 to 16 years and 11 to 14 years respectively. It is succeeded by the third *filling-out* period of adolescence.

In postnatal life there is more than one pattern of tissue growth. The *general pattern* is followed by the bones (except the brain case and sense capsules), the muscles, the organs of respiration, circulation, digestion and excretion and by most external linear dimensions. A *neural pattern* (60 per cent adult size by the age of 2 years and near-adult size by the age of 7 years) is followed by the brain, spinal cord, eyeball, ear and neurocranium. A *thymic pattern* (rapid growth

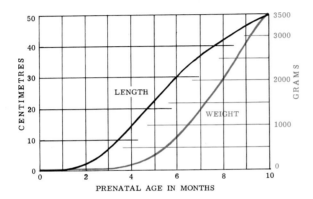

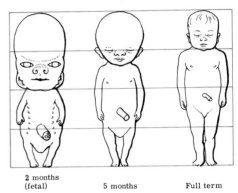

2 months (fetal)　　　5 months　　　Full term

different rates in the two sexes. As a result, the female is relatively precocious, and typically reaches puberty, adolescence and maturity nearly 2 years in advance of the male. *Puberty* has been defined as the period of transition from childhood to adolescence, and is characterized physically by the appearance of secondary sexual characters. It ends, with the onset of ovulation or spermatogenesis, in *adolescence*—the period preceding physical maturity.

If individual children are observed, they show characteristic growth patterns. A regular and probably annual rhythm in increase in height continues until puberty or even later. Superimposed on this are alternating periods of rapid growth and consolidation. The *rapid growth* of the first year is succeeded by slower growth from 1 to 5 years. A second *springing-up* period follows from 5 to 7 years, during which the face and limbs thin, the milk teeth are lost and the brain reaches near-adult size. The second *filling-out* period ends at puberty, when the third and most obvious springing-up period begins and affects all the main tissues except the central nervous system. The intensity, onset and duration of the growth spurt varies between individuals and between boys and

until near puberty and then relative and absolute decrease in size) is followed by the thymus and may be followed by other lymphoid tissues. However, particularly in the tonsils and in the adenoids, growth may be individualized in response to immunological challenges. A *genital pattern* (quiescence from the age of 2 years until puberty and then rapid growth) is followed by the internal and external genitalia.

These gross patterns cannot reveal all the complex and rapid changes of infancy. Far from growing, some organs are reduced in absolute size in the neonatal period. For example, the suprarenal glands and the uterus are both reduced in weight by one-half in the first 2 weeks of life: the suprarenal as its fetal cortex involutes and the uterus as the maternal hormonal stimulus is removed. For some organs (e.g. circulatory), a change of role is involved. For others, a functional level of development is attained. For example, the newborn can cry but not weep since the lacrimal gland does not function until the end of the first month. Of more general features, it may be noted that fat absorption, haemopoiesis and hepatic and renal functions are still immature in infancy.

BODY PROPORTIONS FROM BIRTH TO ADOLESCENCE

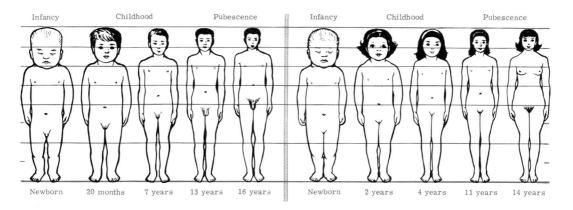

Infancy   Childhood   Pubescence   Infancy   Childhood   Pubescence

Newborn   20 months   7 years   13 years   16 years   Newborn   2 years   4 years   11 years   14 years

PATTERNS OF GROWTH

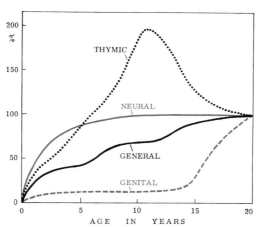

SEX DIFFERENCES IN GROWTH

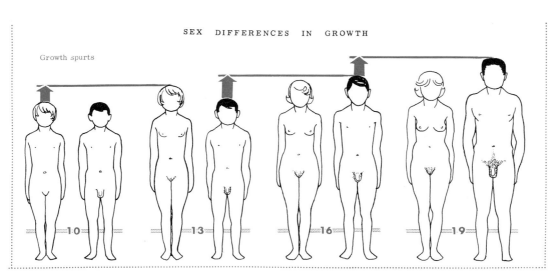

Growth spurts

Early Behavioural Responses

Behavioural activity during development reflects the progressive maturation of the nervous system. The perioral (maxillomandibular) receptors are probably the earliest to develop, and their stimulation evokes the *first reflex* (lateral flexion of the neck away from the stimulated side) in the sixth week of embryonic life. During the next 2 weeks the response spreads as further muscle and nerve fibres become capable of responding. It spreads first to the upper trunk and limb girdle muscles, then to the lower trunk and limb girdle muscles. Until the eighth week this is the only elicitable reflex and can only be elicited from the face. Thereafter, so-called spontaneous movements occur and the total response is largely replaced by *local reflexes* which appear successively in the face, the upper limb, the lower limb and the trunk. The unborn fetus spends periods in *deep sleep*, in *wakefulness* (characterized by responsiveness to stimuli and by apparently purposeful movements) and in *sleep with rapid eye movement* (characterized also by twitching movement and by movement of fluid in and out of the lungs—fetal breathing).

At birth, the tonus of the flexor muscles exceeds that of the anti-gravity muscles, and the resting posture of the newborn is thus a modification of the fetal attitude of generalized flexion. From this posture, the newborn makes spontaneous movements which, for the first week or two, are predominantly random and generalized. Reflexes from the maxillomandibular area are again precociously developed in the newborn. The *search* or *rooting reflex* is a response to perioral touch. At first, repetitive, diminishing, side-to-side movements of the head 'focus' the mouth on the stimulus, but this response is superseded by a single well-directed movement which puts the mouth on the stimulus. If the stimulus is stroked towards the mouth, the lips part and move towards it—the *lip reflex*. The tongue protrudes somewhat and forms a trough which takes the nipple. Stimulation of the lip, front of the tongue, gums or hard palate produces the *sucking reflex* in which the tongue, nipple, areola and surrounding breast are pulled into the mouth. The *swallowing reflex* follows in response to stimulation of the back of the tongue, pharynx, epiglottis or soft palate. Other subcortically mediated reflexes present in the newborn include the *tonic neck reflex* (extension of the limbs on the side towards which the head is turned and flexion of the contralateral limbs—the 'fencing' position), the *startle reflex*, the *grasp reflex* and, usually, an *extensor plantar response*.

After birth the pyramidal, tectospinal and corticopontocerebellar pathways begin to myelinate. During the first month the *vestibular reflexes* become increasingly important in maintaining the posture of the baby's head. At 3 months *retinal postural reflexes* come into play, the corticobulbar fibres in the midbrain begin to myelinate and, soon, the neuromuscular control of the neck is adequate for the child to hold up its head. At 4 months the tonic neck, startle and grasp reflexes can no longer be elicited: integration with the vestibular and retinal reflexes and inhibition by cortical centres has resulted in more complex behaviour patterns. At 6 months all the *superficial reflexes* are present. At 8 months myelination begins in various descending pathways, including corticobulbar (aberrant pyramidal) fibres in the pons and reticulospinal fibres. Presently, maintenance of equilibrium and co-ordination of purposive movements permits standing and crawling. By 1 year the *extensor plantar response* has gradually changed into the adult *flexor* type, and with increasing cortical activity the child soon becomes a walking, talking and thinking being.

The Newborn

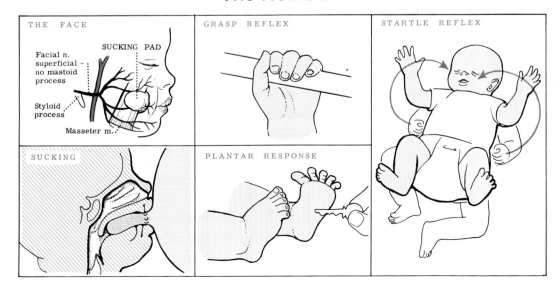

THE FACE — Facial n. superficial – no mastoid process; SUCKING PAD; Styloid process; Masseter m.

SUCKING

GRASP REFLEX

PLANTAR RESPONSE

STARTLE REFLEX

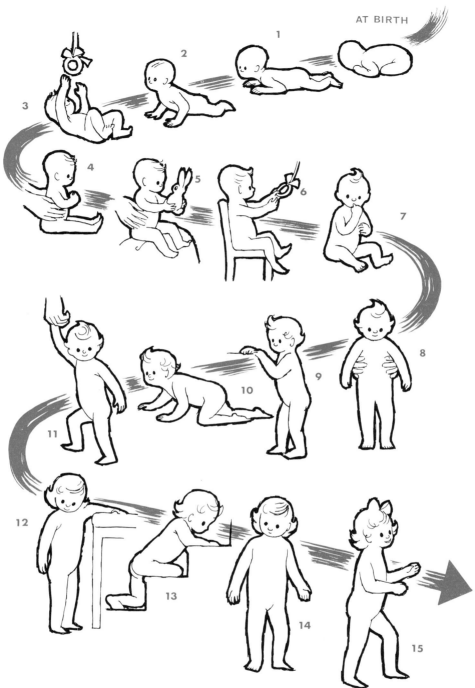

Motor Activities

AT BIRTH	- fetal position	FIVE months	- sit on lap and grasp object
ONE month	- chin up	SIX "	- sit in high chair and grasp
TWO months	- chest up		dangling object
THREE "	- reach and miss	SEVEN "	- sits alone
FOUR "	- sit with support	EIGHT "	- stands with help
		NINE "	- stands holding furniture

TEN months	- crawls	
ELEVEN "	- walks when led	
TWELVE "	- pulls to stand by furniture	
THIRTEEN "	- climbs stairs	
FOURTEEN "	- stands alone	
FIFTEEN "	- walks alone	

Appendix

Organogenesis, Malformations and Deformations

In the preceding pages the sequence of changes within organ systems has been stressed and little attempt has been made to place the changes on a time scale or to relate them to simultaneous changes in other systems. The table on page 169 performs this function for selected stages in organogenesis. It correlates development in the different systems but, as will emerge, has limited value in determining the chronology of malformations. Entries in the table which are unqualified by verbs refer to the first appearance of a particular feature. By interpolating, entries may be used to give an age to intermediate stages and diagrams. Stages before and after those in the table have been considered elsewhere (pp. 64–65 and pp. 162–167).

Since development is progressive, early aberrations will generally produce the most severe terata or malformations. These may result in embryonic or fetal death and absorption, abortion or stillbirth according to the stage at which death occurs. Less severe malformations may permit live birth but be diagnosed as congenital (present from birth) anomalies. The least severe malformations may remain undetected or be discovered incidentally at post-mortem. It has been estimated that terata result in abortion in 20 per cent of all pregnancies, in stillbirth in 2 per cent and in serious congenital anomalies in a further 2 per cent. Since all development, normal and abnormal, results from an interaction between genetic and environmental factors, single factors cannot usually be held responsible for teratogenesis. Nevertheless, in some instances a prime factor may be identified. It has been estimated that in 10 per cent of terata this is a single penetrant gene. In a further 10 per cent a significant maternal condition has been present (infection, fever, diabetes, irradiation, malnutrition, etc.). The remaining 80 per cent are multifactorial.

In many terata (e.g. cleft palate) normal development seems to have been arrested at a certain stage and not completed. Developmental arrest is not, however, the only mechanism which operates, and aberrations of growth and degeneration play their part. An organ such as the lens of the eye may be absent because its primordium never appeared (defective induction, differentiation or growth) or because it appeared and subsequently degenerated. Whatever the mechanism, the final result is determined not only by the primary defect but also by the secondary effects this has on other structures, including disturbances of normal growth processes. The same end result may thus be reached in different ways and from different beginnings. It follows that individual cases and phenocopies and the table of normal development have limited value in determining at what stage a particular malformation may have arisen and less value in determining at what stage the teratogen operated in a particular case.

A distinction can be drawn between *malformations* which arise as a result of errors in morphogenesis and *deformations* which arise later in pregnancy as a result of mechanical forces operating on previously normally formed parts.

In some anomalies (e.g. congenital amputations and ring constrictions of the limbs) strands of tissue—*amniotic bands*—may connect the affected sites with the amnion, and have been held to produce the anomalies by strangulation. However, amniotic bands are also attached to other anomalies where such an explanation is not possible. It seems that amniotic bands are merely adhesions and are secondary to abnormal cell death at the site of their attachment to the fetus.

Mechanical forces are more certainly involved in the group of anomalies termed the *congenital postural deformities*. The most common and important conditions in this group are the various forms of *talipes* (club foot), *congenital sternomastoid torticollis* (wry neck), *congenital postural scoliosis* (curvature of the spine) and *congenital dislocation of the hip*. It also includes other limb and craniofacial anomalies, including the *compression facies*. These conditions appear to be produced by compression within the uterus as the fetus continues to grow and the volume of the amniotic fluid decreases in absolute terms. Individual conditions in the group commonly occur in association with each other and with primigravidity, maternal hypertension, oligohydramnios, breech presentation and fetal growth retardation. Experimentally they occur in rats in which oligohydramnios has been produced by amniocentesis. Renal agenesis in a fetus usually produces oligohydramnios, pulmonary hypoplasia and congenital postural deformities. However, if a fetus with renal agenesis shares the same amniotic sac as its normal twin, none of these secondary conditions is produced. The factors involved in congenital postural deformities are not solely environmental. For example, congenital dislocation of the hip is also associated with joint laxity (a monogenic effect) and with acetabular deficiency (a polygenic effect). At birth the incidence of simple postural deformities is higher than that of malformations. However, unlike malformations, many postural deformities correct spontaneously and most others respond to early postural assistance.

Chronology of prenatal organogenesis

Period	Stage					
Pre-embryonic	3rd week	Cardiogenic area heart tubes form	oral membrane; head-fold will enclose foregut	neural plate; groove	intraembryonic mesoderm	cloacal membrane tail-fold will enclose hindgut
Embryonic	4th week	Heart tubes fuse and loop	oral membrane ruptures; laryngo-tracheal groove; pharyngeal pouches; thyroid rudiment; Rathke's pouch; hepatic diverticulum	neural tube closes primary brain vesicles; cervical flexure; neural crest segments; optic vesicles; lens placodes; otic placodes–vesicles	limb buds	nephrogenic cord—nephric ducts
Embryonic	5th week	Septum primum; atrioventricular cushions	nasal placodes tongue primordia; lung buds; tubo-tympanic recesses; pancreatic diverticula	midbrain flexure; spinal nerve roots; optic cups; lens vesicles	joint flexures; hands and feet	nephric ducts reach cloaca; ureteric buds reach metanephric blastemata; genital ridges; urorectal septum; genital tubercle
Embryonic	6th week	Ostium primum closes; aortico-pulmonary septation; cardiac muscle; haemopoiesis in liver	dental laminae; palatal processes; primitive nasal septum; oronasal membrane ruptures; pleuropericardial openings close; midgut loop herniates caecum/appendix; spleen	pontine flexure; cerebral hemispheres; nerve plexuses; cerebellum	chondrification; intramembranous ossification	Müllerian ducts; urethral plate
Embryonic	7th week	Interventricular septum complete		choroid plexus; eyelid folds	skeletal muscle; fingers and toes	metanephric vesicles; distinctive testes/ovaries; cloacal membrane breaks down
Embryonic	8th week		enamel organs; external nares plugged; bronchioles; pleuroperitoneal canals close; smooth muscle		smooth muscle; endochondral ossification	Müllerian ducts fuse; smooth muscle
Fetal	3rd month	Haemopoiesis in bone marrow	nasal septum and palate fusion complete; midgut loop returns	eyelids fuse		testes near future internal ring; processus vaginalis; distinctive external genitalia
Fetal	Months 4–7		pulmonary alveoli (6)	myelination (4); pupillary membrane ruptures (7); eyelids separate (7)		vaginal plate (4) canalizes (5); testes in inguinal canal (7)

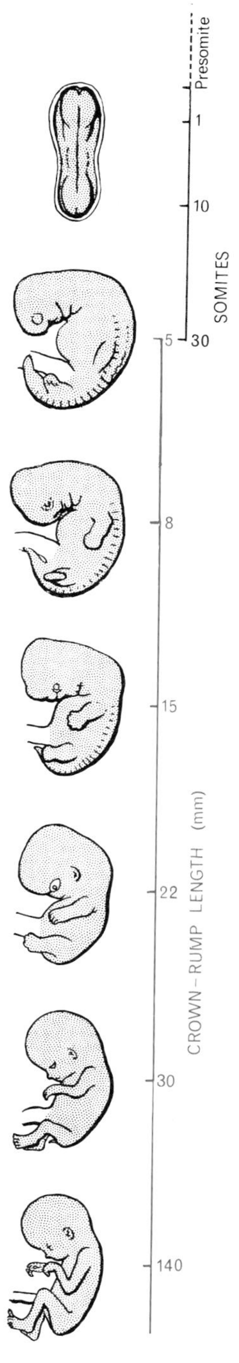

Presomite
1
10
SOMITES
30
5
8
15
22
CROWN–RUMP LENGTH (mm)
30
140

Index

Duct/s (*contd*)
lacrimal, 144
lymphatic, 156
Müllerian (paramesonephric), 92–3, **96–7**, 99–101, 169
nasolacrimal, 68
nephric, 94–5, 169
of epididymis, 35–6, 96–7
of Gartner, 97
pancreatic, 86–7
papillary (Bellini), 94
paraurethral, 98
parotid, 74
semicircular, 145
submandibular, 74
thoracic, 156
thyroglossal, 78–9
urogenital, 29
vitellointestinal, 54–7, 89; *see also* Stalk, of yolk sac
Wolffian (mesonephric), 92–100, 154
Ductule
aberrant, of testis, 96–7
efferent, of epididymis, 34–5, 96
Ductus
arteriosus, 146, **154–5**, 158–9
persistent, 160–1
deferens (vas), **32**, 36–7, 92–3, **96–7**
venosus, 156–9
Duodenum, 82–3, 86–90
Dysgenesis, ovarian, 16
Dysostosis, craniocleidal, 116–17

Ear
external, 65–6, **69**, 73, 131, 145, 162
internal, 64, 131, **145**, 164
middle, 66, 78–9, **145**, 163
Early pregnancy factor (EPF), 46
Ectoderm, **7**, 28, 30, 48, 50, **52**, 56, 65–6, 72, 78, 82–3, 88, 98–9, 102, 104, 112, 118–20, 122–5
extraembryonic, 50, 52
Ectopia
ovarii, 100
testis, 100
vesicae (exstrophy of bladder), 100–1
Egg, *see also* Ovum
mediolecithal, 28–9
megalecithal, 28–30
miolecithal, 28–30
Ejaculation, 36
Embryo
age estimation, **64–5**, 102, 169
developmental levels, 6, **64–5**, 169
dimensions, 64–5, 169
general development, **52–7**, 64–5
nutrition of, 58–63, 162
Eminence, hypobranchial, *see* Copula
Emission, 36
Endoderm, **7**, 24, 28, 30, 48, **51–7**, 66, 72, 76, 78, 82–3, 88, 90, 94, 96, 98–9
extraembryonic, 50, 52
Endometrium, 32–3, 38, **42–4**, 46–7, 50
Endorphins, β, 60
Epiblast, 50–2, 96
Epidermis, 24–5, 72, 102, **118–19**

Epididymis, 34–7, 96–7
appendages of, 96–7
head, 34
tail, 36
Epiglottis, **76–7**, 131, 166
Epiphysis, 108–9, 111
Epispadias, 100–1
Epitrichium, 118–19
Eponychium, 118–19
Epoophoron, 97
Exomphalos, 91
Eye, 56, 65–6, 68–9, 130, 133, **144**, 162, 164, 168

Face, 65–9, 73, 75, 102, 164–6
anomalies, 80–1
Facies, compression, 100, 168
Fertilization, 6–7, 14, 26, 32, **46**, 50, 58, 92, 96
Fertility, 36
Fetus, 6, 44, 48, 64, 120, 144, 146, 148, 158, **162**, 164–6, 168–9
viable, 162
Fin, nasal, 70–1, 80
Fingerprints, 21, 112
Fishes, 48, 66, 72
Fissure
choroid, of eye, 144
oral, 69, 73
petrotympanic, 74
Fistula
branchial, 73, 80–1
cloacal, 91, 101
tracheo-oesophageal, 80–1, 91
rectal, 101
umbilical, 91
Flexures, of nervous system, 54, 65, **132–3**, 169
Fluid
amniotic (liquor), **56**, 94, 118, 142, 163, 166, 168
cerebrospinal (CSF), **126**, 142
Fold/s
aryepiglottic, 76–7
genital, 92–3, 98–9
head, 48–9, **54–7**, 64, 82–4, 149, 169
inguinal, 99
lateral, 48–9, **54–7**, 64, 84
nail, 118–19
peritoneal, anomalous, 91
tail, 48–9, **54–7**, 64, 82–4, 96, 98, 169
Follicle
hair, 118–19
ovarian, 32, **38–41**, 58, 96–7
thyroid, 78
Fontanelles, 163
Foot, club (talipes equinovarus), 116–17, 168
Foramen/foramina
caecum, 76–9
epiploic (aditus to lesser sac), 87–9
interventricular, 150–4
of skull, 106–7
ovale, 146, **152–3**, 158–9, 160–1
Fornices, vaginal, 38, 97
Fossa
incisive, 70, 80
nasal, 68–71

Gall bladder, 90–1
Gamete, **7**, 15, 16–18, 32, 82
Gametocyte, 15, 17
Gametogenesis, 7, **14–15**, 18–19, 26, 32
Ganglion/ganglia, 122
autonomic, 123, 125–8
of cranial nerves, 70, 73, 122–3, **125–8**, 145
parasympathetic, 125–8
spinal, 122–3, 125–7
sympathetic, 78–9, 125–7
Gastrula/gastrulation, 7, **23–4**, 28–9
Gelatinoreticulum (cardiac jelly), 149–50
Genes, 9, **14**, 18–19, 21, 96, 100, 168
loci, 18, 21
regulator, 14
structural, 14
Genitalia, external, 92–3, **98–9**, 164, 169
anomalies, 100–1
Genome, **14**, 16, 26
Genotype, **16**, 18–19, 22
heterozygous, 18–19
homozygous, 18–19
Germ layers, 6–7, 23
Gestation, 6, 42, **44**, 59
Glands
bulbourethral, 36–7, **97**, 99
endocrine, 66–7, **78–9**, 162
endometrial, 38, **42–3**, 46, 58–9
intestinal, 88
lacrimal, 130, 144
mammary, 40, **118–19**, 162–4, 166
oral, 73, 130
parathyroid, 78–80
paraurethral, 97–8
parenchyma of, 66
parotid, 73, 130
pineal, 132, 134–5
pituitary, *see* Hypophysis cerebri
prostate, 32, 36–7, **98–9**
salivary, 74, 130
sebaceous, 118–19
stroma of, 66
sublingual, 74, 130
submandibular, 74, 130
suprarenal, 54, **78–80**, 94, 99, 125, 163–4
sweat, 118–19
thymus, 66, **78–80**, 148, 163–5
thyroid, 67, **76–81**, 163, 169
urethral, 36, 98–9
uterine, 38; *see also* Glands, endometrial
vestibular, 97–8
Glans
clitoridis, 98
penis, 98–9
Glioblast, 124
Glomerulus, 94–5
Gonad, 29, 34, 38, 54, 56, 92–3, **96**, 99, 164
anomalies, 100
descent, 99–100
Gonadotrophins
human chorionic (hCG), **41**, 60, 62
pituitary, 40–1, 44

Phylogeny, 7
Pit, olfactory, 66, **68**, 106
Placenta, 6, 30–1, 41, 44, 48, 50, **58–63**, 146, 158–9, 162
  anomalies, 62–3
  chorioallantoic, 30–1, 62
  choriovitelline (yolk sac), 30–1
  haemochorial, 62
  inverted yolk sac, 30–1
  labyrinthine, 59–62
  placenta praevia, 62–3
  uterine, sites of, 62–3
  villous, 59, 62
Placode, 56
  epibranchial, **73**, 125, 128
  lens, 56, **144**, 169
  nasal, 66, **68**, 125, 128, 169
  otic, 64–5, 128, **145**, 169
Plate
  basal, 58–60
  cortical, 128, 134
  chorionic, 58, 60
  epiphyseal, 108–9
  neural, 24, 48–9, 54–6, 64, 68, **122–5**, 169
  notochordal, 52–3, 124
  prechordal, **50–3**, 64, 104
  urethral, 98–9, 169
  vaginal, **96–8**, 101, 169
Pleura, 82–3
Poles
  animal and vegetative, 23, 25, 28, 39, 46
  embryonic and abembryonic, 50–1, 58
Polydactyly, 116–17
Polyembryony, 44
Polymorphism
  balanced, 20
  genetic, 20
Polyspermy, 46
Pouch
  coelomic, 29
  pharyngeal, 56–7, 66, 72, 76, **78–80**, 145, 169
  Rathké's, 67, **70–1**, 125, 128, 169
Pregnancy, extrauterine (ectopic), 62–3
Prepuce, 99, 163
Primitive, 24
Process
  costal, 104–5
  dentinal, 120
  notochordal, 52–3, 64
  palatal, 66, **70–1**, 80, 169
  styloid, 74
Processus vaginalis, 99–100, 169
Progesterone, 32–3, **40–4**, 48, 60, 62, 118, 162
Prolactin (PRL), **40**, 60, 118
  inhibiting factor (PIF), **40**, 60
Proliferation, cellular, 9, **24**, 26, 50, 78
Prominence
  facial, 66, **68–71**, 80, 106, 108, 125
  frontonasal, **66–71**, 80, 131
  mandibular, 64, 66, **68–9**, 71–2, 106, 131
  maxillary, 66, **68–72**, 80–1, 106, 131

nasal
  lateral, 68, 106
  medial, 68
  premaxillary, 68, **70**, 80–1, 106
Pronephros, 94–5
Pronucleus, 7, 46
Prosencephalon (forebrain), 122–3, 128–9, **132–9**
Prostaglandins, 62, 162
Pseudohermaphroditism, 100
Pseudopregnancy, 44
Puberty, 6, 44, 118, **164**
Puerperium, 44

Radiation, ionizing, 26
Reaction
  decidual, **46**, 58, 62
  precidual, **42**
Recess
  dorsal and ventral, of pharyngeal pouches, 78–9
  hepatoenteric, 86–8
  pancreaticoenteric, 86–8
  pneumatoenteric, 86–8
  tubotympanic, **78–9**, 145, 169
Rectum, 88, 92–5
Reflexes, 162–3, 166
Replication, 9, **12**, 124
Repressor, Müllerian, 96
Reproduction, asexual and sexual, 7
Reptiles, 28, 30
Respiratory system, 48, 57, 66–7, **76–7**, 82–5, 146, 158–9, 162–4
Rete
  ovarii, 96–7
  testis, 34–5, 96
Reticulum
  mesenchymatous, 50–1
  stellate, 120–1
Rhesus incompatibility, 60
Rhombencephalon (hindbrain), 122–3, 128–33
Rib, cervical, 116–17
Ribonucleic acids (RNA), 9, 12
Ridge/s
  apical, of limb bud, 112
  bulbar, 150–2
  friction, 112
  genital, 95–6, 169
  milk, 118–19
  neural, 54, 68, **70–1**, 122–5
Rodents, 7
Rubella (viruses), 26, 60, 144, 145

Sac
  aortic, 72, 78, **150**, 154
  dental, 120
  endolymphatic, 145
  hypophyseal, 70
  infundibular, 70
  lymph, 156
  nasal, 68–71
  nasolacrimal, 68
  pleural, 84
  yolk, 30–1, **47–58**, 60, 84–5, 88–91, 96, 146–9
Sclerotome, 104–6, 126
Segmentation, metameric, 29, 54–7, **104**
Semen, 32, 36

Septum
  aorticopulmonary, **150–3**, 160, 169
  bulbar, 152
  cotyledonary, 59–61
  nasal, **69–71**, 106–7, 162, 169
  primum, 150–3, 169
  secundum, 152–3
  sinuatrial, 150
  transversum, **52–7**, 84, 86, 90, 94, 149–50
  urorectal, 82–3, **88**, 91–5, 98, 101, 169
  ventricular, 150–3, 161
Sex, determination, 7, **15**, 46, 92, 96
Sheath
  perichordal, 104–5
  root, 120–1
Shell, trophoblastic, 58–60
Sinus
  aortic, 150–2
  cervical, 73
  coronary, 152, 156–8
  lateral cervical (branchial), 80–1
  of pericardium, 153
  paranasal, 70, 163
  pre-auricular, 80
  sinus venosus, 149–52
  urachal, 100
  urogenital, 94–100
  venous of dura mater, 126, 154–5
Situs inversus, **27**, 91, 160
Skeleton, **104–11**, 114–15, 125, 163
Skin, 102, 104, **118–19**, 125, 131
Skull, 29, 102, **106–9**, 122
  anomalies, 116–17, 142–3
  moulding, 163
  newborn, 163
Smoking, 26
Somatomammotropin, human chorionic (hCS), 60
Somatopleure, **30–1**, 51, 54, 84, 112, 126–7
Somites, 24–5, 54–7, 64, 74–5, 94–5, **102–6**, 112, 114, 118, 169
Space
  intervillous, 58–61
  labyrinthine, 58, 60
  perilymphatic, 145
  perivitelline, 46
  subarachnoid, 126
Spermatid, 34–5
Spermatocyte, 15, 34–5
Spermatogenesis, 7, **34–6**, 40, 164
Spermatogonium, 15, **34–5**, 96
Spermatozoa (sperm), 6, 7, 9, 32, **34–6**, 46, 47, 92
Spina bifida, 116, 142–3
Spindle
  achromatic, **14–5**, 47, 51
  maturation, 39, 46–7
Splanchnopleure, **30–1**, 51, 54, 126–7
Spleen, 86–7, 169
Stabilizer, Wolffian, 96
Stalk
  connecting (body), 30, 48, 50, **52–3**, 84, 146, 149
  of yolk sac, 84, **88**, 91
Stem, villous, 58–9